Sex

BOOKS BY VERNON COLEMAN

The Medicine Men (1975)
Paper Doctors (1976)
Everything You Want To Know About Ageing (1976)
Stress Control (1978)
The Home Pharmacy (1980)
Aspirin or Ambulance (1980)
Face Values (1981)
Guilt (1982)
The Good Medicine Guide (1982)
Stress And Your Stomach (1983)
Bodypower (1983)
An A to Z Of Women's Problems (1984)
Bodysense (1984)
Taking Care Of Your Skin (1984)
A Guide to Child Health (1984)
Life Without Tranquillisers (1985)
Diabetes (1985)
Arthritis (1985)
Eczema and Dermatitis (1985)
The Story Of Medicine (1985, 1998)
Natural Pain Control (1986)
Mindpower (1986)
Addicts and Addictions (1986)
Dr Vernon Coleman's Guide To Alternative Medicine (1988)
Stress Management Techniques (1988)
Overcoming Stress (1988)
Know Yourself (1988)
The Health Scandal (1988)
The 20 Minute Health Check (1989)
Sex For Everyone (1989)
Mind Over Body (1989)
Eat Green Lose Weight (1990)
Why Animal Experiments Must Stop (1991)
The Drugs Myth (1992)
How To Overcome Toxic Stress (1991)
Why Doctors Do More Harm Than Good (1993)
Stress and Relaxation (1993)
Complete Guide To Sex (1993)
How to Conquer Backache (1993)

Betrayal of Trust (1994)
How to Conquer Pain (1994)
Know Your Drugs (1994, 1997)
Food for Thought (1994)
The Traditional Home Doctor (1994)
I Hope Your Penis Shrivels Up (1994)
People Watching (1995)
Relief from IBS (1995)
The Parent's Handbook (1995)
Oral Sex: Bad Taste And Hard To Swallow? (1995)
Why Is Pubic Hair Curly? (1995)
Men in Dresses (1996)
Power over Cancer (1996)
Crossdressing (1996)
How To Get The Best Out Of Prescription Drugs (1996)
How To Get The Best Out of Alternative Medicine (1996)
How To Conquer Arthritis (1996)
High Blood Pressure (1996)
How To Stop Your Doctor Killing You (1996)
Fighting For Animals (1996)
Alice and Other Friends (1996)
Dr Coleman's Fast Action Health Secrets (1997)
Dr Vernon Coleman's Guide to Vitamins and Minerals (1997)
Spiritpower (1997)
Other People's Problems (1998)
How To Publish Your Own Book (1999)
How To Relax and Overcome Stress (1999)
Animal Rights – Human Wrongs (1999)
Superbody (1999)
The 101 Sexiest, Craziest, Most Outrageous
   Agony Column Questions (and Answers) of All Time (1999)
Strange but True (2000)
How To Make Money While Watching TV (2000)
Food for Thought [revised edition] (2000)
Daily Inspirations (2000)
Stomach Problems: Relief At Last (2001)
How To Overcome Guilt (2001)
Animal Rights – Human Wrongs Pocket Edition (2001)

reports

Prostate Trouble (2000)
Vitamins and Minerals (2000)

How To Campaign (2000)
Genetic Engineering (2000)
Osteoporosis (2000)
Vaccines (2000)
Alternative Medicine (2000)

novels

The Village Cricket Tour (1990)
The Bilbury Chronicles (1992)
Bilbury Grange (1993)
Mrs Caldicot's Cabbage War (1993)
Bilbury Revels (1994)
Deadline (1994)
The Man Who Inherited a Golf Course (1995)
Bilbury Country (1996)
Second Innings (1999)
Around the Wicket (2000)
It's Never Too Late (2001)

short stories

Bilbury Pie (1995)

on cricket

Thomas Winsden's Cricketing Almanack (1983)
Diary Of A Cricket Lover (1984)

as Edward Vernon

Practice Makes Perfect (1977)
Practise What You Preach (1978)
Getting Into Practice (1979)
Aphrodisiacs – An Owner's Manual (1983)
Aphrodisiacs – An Owner's Manual (Turbo Edition) (1984)
The Complete Guide To Life (1984)

as Marc Charbonnier

Tunnel (novel 1980)

with Alice

Alice's Diary (1989)
Alice's Adventures (1992)

with Dr Alan C Turin

No More Headaches (1981)

Sex

Things Your Mother Never Told You
(And You Never Dared Ask Her)

Vernon Coleman

European Medical Journal

Published by European Medical Journal, Publishing House, Trinity Place, Barnstaple, Devon EX32 9HJ, England.

This book is copyright. Enquiries should be addressed to the author c/o the publishers.

© Vernon Coleman 2001. The right of Vernon Coleman to be identified as the author of this work has been asserted in accordance with the Copyright, Designs and Patents Act 1988.

ISBN: 1 898947 29 5

All rights reserved. No part may be reproduced, stored in a retrieval system or transmitted, in any form or by any means, electronic, mechanical, photocopying, recording or otherwise without the prior written permission of the author and publisher. This book is sold subject to the condition that it shall not by way of trade or otherwise be lent, re-sold, hired out or otherwise circulated without the publisher's prior consent in any form of binding or cover other than that in which it is published.

A catalogue record for this book is available from the British Library.

Printed by J.W. Arrowsmith Ltd., Bristol

Warning

This book is not intended to be, and cannot be, an alternative to personal, professional, medical advice.

Readers should immediately consult a trained and properly qualified health professional, whom they trust and respect, for advice about any symptom or health problem which requires diagnosis, treatment or any kind of medical attention.

While the advice and information in this book are believed to be accurate at the time of going to press, neither the author nor the publisher can accept any legal responsibility for errors or omissions which may be made.

To Donna Antoinette Coleman, the Welsh Princess

~ Sex ~

Afterplay

When a man has ejaculated his interest in sex (and his partner) may decline rapidly. As his penis shrinks so goes his sex drive. Many men fall asleep as soon as they have had an orgasm and this is a physiological consequence of sex rather than a comment or an insult. The human sexual urges were designed for procreation and when a man has ejaculated his purpose is done – if he remains sexually interested he will be more likely to hinder than to help the process of conception.

Women are quite different. They remain alert, sensitive and loving after intercourse. Many say that their need for love and reassurance and comfort is greater after sex than at any other time. They are likely to feel lonely and abandoned and depressed and 'used' if their partner rolls over and falls asleep the minute he has ejaculated.

This problem can to a certain extent be alleviated by making love in the morning when both partners are wide awake rather than at night when both are tired (and he is, therefore, more likely to fall asleep anyway).

And women should remember that men are more vulnerable and more sensitive than they appear to be. Rushing off to the bathroom after making love will not do his ego much good. Keep a towel or box of tissues nearby if you want to avoid the inevitable

---

The most popular sexual position is the missionary position – generally favoured by 60% of adults.

damp patch on the sheets. And be careful not to say anything that could be construed as critical. If you want to talk avoid household problems and concentrate on romantic plans and aspirations for the future. Remember, too, that just as women like to be told how much they are loved so men like to be told how wonderful they are in bed.

ANAL SEX

Although anal sex is illegal in many parts of the world it is remarkably popular among heterosexuals. One in ten heterosexual couples regularly have anal sex and more than half of heterosexuals have tried it.

Anal sex first became popular as a means of avoiding conception.

Today, however, most couples who practise anal sex do so because they find it exciting. Men claim that penetrating a tight anal sphincter gives them a special type of pleasure while women who like anal sex say either that they get a more intense orgasm or that they enjoy the feeling of being dominated and that they like the excitement of something which they think of as being forbidden.

Because anal sex may be painful it tends to appeal to men who like to be dominant and women who like to be submissive – though with the aid of a vibrator it is, of course, possible for a woman to take the dominant role. Anal sex is the only way a woman can 'penetrate' a man.

If you want to try anal sex remember that lubrication is vital. There is little natural lubrication and the sphincter which guards the rectum is very tight.

The 'active' partner should start by gently pushing a finger tip into the 'passive' partner's anus, pressing very gently. The 'pas-

---

An Italian man suffocated to death between the 48FF size breasts of his mistress.

---

sive' partner should bear down on the finger tip. It may help to tighten up the anal sphincter and then to let it relax. Once the sphincter is opened and well lubricated penetration with a penis or vibrator can commence. The lubrication should be spread over the anus and the penis or vibrator. The anal sphincter normally closes automatically when any object approaches from outside so the active partner will need a considerable amount of determination to overcome this natural barrier. The passive partner should try hard to relax.

You are unlikely to be able to penetrate very far on your first attempts.

Various sexual positions are suitable for anal intercourse. Any of the rear entry positions will do but the standard ('doggy' style) rear entry position is probably the most popular. It is possible to have anal intercourse in the traditional face to face missionary position though she may need to open her legs and pull her knees up towards her chest to make this possible. It is possible for either or both partners to reach an orgasm when making love in this position.

Now some warnings.

First, anal sex is illegal in some parts of the world and even attempting it in private with a consenting partner may result in criminal proceedings if you are discovered.

Second, anal intercourse is often painful – particularly the first time. It is likely to be especially painful if the passive partner has piles or any other anal condition.

Third, if anal and vaginal intercourse are mixed, infection is a real hazard. There is a risk that bacteria from the intestinal tract may be introduced into the vagina. To avoid this risk vaginal sex should not follow anal sex until the penis has been cleaned. If a condom is used (which it should be, of course) then you should change condoms when changing entrances.

A woman living in the south of England claims to have had sex in 22 different makes of car.

Fourth, – and this warning is extremely important – I don't believe that there is much doubt that anal intercourse is a major factor in the development of the disorder usually known as AIDS.

Although the medical establishment defines AIDS as a specific disease I'm not even sure that it exists, but, whatever the truth may be, there does seem to be evidence confirming that anal sex increases the risk of this problem developing. And the risks may be dramatically increased if you practise this type of sex with a partner who is a needle using drug addict or with a partner who is bisexual. I believe that the risks are also dramatically increased if you have anal sex with more than one partner or with a partner who is promiscuous. It is of course possible to transmit other infections when having sex this way. A condom will provide some protection. It is sensible to use a strong condom when using this entrance.

Fifth, regular anal sex can lead to stretching of the anal sphincter. And this could lead to incontinence.

Aphrodisiacs

Clothes are probably the best and most effective aphrodisiac. Most men are turned on by black stockings, high-heeled shoes, uplift bras, garter belts, skin-tight trousers and sweaters, low-cut dresses, flimsy night wear and so on. And most women are turned on by the knowledge that they are turning men on.

But a number of comestibles are reputed to have aphrodisiac qualities. Here is an appraisal of some of the best known:

Amyl Nitrate
Amyl nitrate increases the blood supply to various parts of the body and can make an individual feel more excited but there are real dangers with this substance and it is not safe for use as an aphrodisiac. Some users claim that if you break an ampoule

---

A survey of people who put personal advertisements in magazines showed that 73% were looking purely for sex.

---

of amyl nitrate and inhale the fumes you will feel a rush of sexual excitement.

It is also claimed that the drug helps to relax the anal sphincter (making it popular with homosexuals and heterosexuals wanting to try anal sex) but the hazards outweigh any value it may have. Definitely not recommended.

Alcohol
In large quantities alcohol may increase desire but diminish performance. It certainly can cause impotence in men and frigidity in women. If taken in small quantities alcohol can be an aphrodisiac – releasing inhibitions and suppressing fears and anxieties. Alcohol works as an aphrodisiac in two ways. It depresses the restrictive control centres in the brain and thereby allows desires which are normally suppressed to surface. In addition it causes a general dilatation of the body's superficial blood vessels and produces a generalised skin glow. For most people one and a half to two glasses of wine are enough – more will cause problems. Alcohol usually begins to produce a result about fifteen minutes after it has been drunk. If food is consumed at the same time the rate at which the alcohol is absorbed into the blood stream slows down. Soda water increases this rate but reduces the length of time that the effect lasts. The best type of alcohol is probably champagne – because of the romantic associations. But some experts claim that green Chartreuse is an excellent aphrodisiac.

Chocolate
Since the nineteenth century chocolate has been regarded as a sexual stimulant and given as a love token. Chocolate contains phenylethylamine – a substance related to the amphetamines – which is the 'love chemical' which helps us fall in love.

If you're looking for a man with a high sex drive then look for one with a deep voice.

Foods

Figs have a sexy reputation because some people think they look like the vulva of a woman. Cucumbers, bananas, carrots and other similarly shaped foods have a reputation for being sexy because of their phallic shape. The avocado pear has a reputation as an aphrodisiac because it is the same sort of shape as a woman's womb. (The Aztecs had such a high regard for the aphrodisiac qualities of the avocado that they kept all their virgins indoors during the avocado season). Some foods have a sexy reputation because of their smell. So, foods with a 'musky' odour such as asparagus, artichokes, truffles and mushrooms are regarded as aphrodisiacs. Louis XIV's mistress spiced up the old king's love life with asparagus hollandaise, prepared from eggs and asparagus. Caviare got its reputation as an aphrodisiac through Rasputin the Russian monk. The long-established association between oysters and sex is difficult to explain, although oysters do contain chemicals related to sex hormones. Some users claim that the opening oyster shell reminds them of a woman.

Ginseng

Ginseng gained its reputation because of its phallic shaped root. But the evidence does not support the reputation. Definitely not recommended.

Magic Mushrooms

Psilocybe and amanita, obtained from two allegedly sexually potent magic mushrooms, are sometimes used separately and sometimes together. Amanita is said to give those who use it great energy and staying power. Some experimenters have reported that it produces forceful and unnaturally prolonged orgasms with repeated ejaculations and violent vaginal contrac-

---

One in 10 teenage couples have sex on a first date if neither drink alcohol. If both drink alcohol, one in five teenage couples have sex on their first date.

tions. It also distorts the processes of thought and can produce terrifying results. Psilocybe has far less dramatic sexual effects but has a chemical structure quite similar to that of LSD and is, therefore, a hallucinogenic drug. Magic mushrooms are definitely not recommended.

Marijuana
Marijuana removes inhibitions (in the same way that alcohol does) but has no direct, stimulating sexual effect. Indeed, some evidence suggests that marijuana may lower the amount of circulating testosterone. Definitely not recommended.

Mescaline
Mescaline is reputed to have aphrodisiac qualities but it is also a powerful hallucinogenic and people who use it may have frightening 'trips'. It is also reputed to be extremely addictive. Definitely not recommended.

Prescribed Drugs
Some prescribed drugs can produce impotence. It is reputed that other prescribed drugs may increase sexual appetite. One doctor reported that a forty year old woman took an appetite suppressant and found that her sexual appetite rose so much that her husband had to take another job nearer to home so that he could call in at lunchtime to satisfy his wife's greatly increased sexual demands.

Rhinoceros Horn
Powdered rhinoceros horn acquired its reputation as an aphrodisiac because of its phallic shape. Definitely not recommended.

> Teenage pupils in the United States who have already had sex have been told that they can consider themselves 'secondary virgins' if they stop doing it.

Spanish Fly

Spanish fly is a powder derived from the cantharis beetle which is found in southern Europe. The beetles are anaesthetised, dried and then heated until they disintegrate into powder. Spanish fly has a reputation as an aphrodisiac but it can cause internal bleeding and can kill. Definitely not recommended.

Vitamin E

Vitamin E originally earned its massive reputation as an aphrodisiac on the basis of a limited amount of research work done on rat fertility patterns. I have been unable to find any clinical evidence to prove that humans can improve their sexual prowess or performance by taking vitamin E.

Yohimbine

Yohimbine, from the yohimbe tree, does increase the flow of blood to the sexual organs and also increases nervous activity in that area. But people who have tried it claim that the effect is purely genital and there is no accompanying sense of pleasure or satisfaction. Definitely not recommended.

BABIES: HOW TO CHOOSE THE SEX OF YOUR COMING BABY

Over the centuries many people have tried to find ways to manipulate the odds and to choose the sex of their baby.

- The ancient Greeks believed that sperm from the left testicle produced a girl while sperm from the right testicle would produce a boy. In order to try to choose the sex of their next baby Greek fathers would have one testicle temporarily tied off.
- French noblemen were even more determined to obtain male

> Couples between the ages of 21 and 25 tend to have sex more often than at any other age.

~ Sex ~

heirs. They would sometimes have their left testicles cut off completely.
- In Austria women giving birth who wanted a son the next time would ask the midwife to bury the placenta or afterbirth underneath the nearest nut tree.
- Women living on the Pelew Islands, east of the Philippines in the Pacific Ocean, used to dress up in their partners clothes in the belief that this would help ensure that they had a baby boy.

Popular theories seem to emerge all over the world.

One modern idea popular in several countries is that if a man wants a boy he should make sure that he throws his underpants down on the right hand side of the bed before making love to his partner.

Other widespread theories designed to ensure the birth of a baby boy include:

- making love with your shoes on
- eating a raw egg beforehand
- making love only when the wind is coming from the North

These days scientists try to be more logical when advising parents on the best ways to choose the sex of their babies. I do not recommend (let alone guarantee) any of this information but here is some available information:

1. If you want a boy make love on the day of ovulation. If you want a girl make love at least two days before ovulation – the time when the female egg is released. Ovulation usually occurs twelve to sixteen days before a menstrual bleed starts. One in seven women feel a pain when they ovulate.
2. If you want a girl wait until you are older. Young couples seem to have more sons. Older parents seem to be more likely to give birth to daughters.

Most men have their first ejaculation at the age of 14.

3. If you want a boy make love during a war. There is a rise in the number of boys born during or just after a war.
4. If you have a string of sons and are desperate for a daughter keep trying – the odds are getting better. The more children you have the more likely you are to have a girl.
5. Women who want a girl should either marry an anaesthetist or a fighter pilot. Both groups seem to father more girls than boys.
6. Eat lots of vegetables (but no lettuce, raw cabbage or cauliflower, spinach or cress) and lots of fresh fruit if you want a boy. If you want a girl keep your consumption of salt low but drink plenty of milk and eat lots of rice and pasta.

Celibacy

If you haven't made love for a while then your sex drive will fall.

If you haven't had sex for several months then your natural sexual urges will gradually become weaker and weaker.

People who are celibate (either through choice or because they are separated from their partner or because they cannot find a suitable partner) often find that as time goes by their interest in sex falls.

There is a simple physical explanation for what may seem to be an alarming phenomenon.

If you haven't had sex for a while then the quantity of sex hormones circulating in your body will fall. Eventually the level will fall so low that your interest in and enthusiasm for sex will also fall.

Once you start having sex again your circulating sex hormone levels will rise – and then you'll gradually recover your interest in sex.

The largest penis ever measured was 13 inches long.

Cervical Cap

Looks like a large thimble and fits over the cervix to prevent sperm passing out of the vagina and into the womb. Because it was invented by a doctor from Holland it is sometimes known as a Dutch Cap. The main advantage of the cervical cap over the condom is that it doesn't interfere with anyone's pleasure. The main disadvantage is that it doesn't provide much protection against infection. It is fairly easy to pop a cap into position. If put in during a menstrual period it will temporarily halt the flow of blood. Custom built cervical caps are now available which contain a one way valve and which can be left in position for months at a time. The valve allows menstrual fluid to flow out but doesn't allow sperm to get in.

The cervix and uterus (or womb)

At the top end of the vagina can be felt the cervix or neck of the womb.

The womb itself is hollow and shaped rather like an upside down pear – with the cervix where the pear stalk would be. The uterus consists of extremely strong muscles which can stretch to many times their normal size for months at a time during pregnancy and then revert back to their original size afterwards.

Every month the womb lining develops in order to provide a nourishing site for any egg which may be fertilized, giving it a chance to develop into a foetus. Since the womb is tucked well away inside a woman's body any developing baby will be protected by thick muscle and hard bone. The lining of the uterus, the endometrium, is under the control of hormones and the bleeding which marks the end of each menstrual cycle is a result of the endometrium breaking down and being discharged from the uterus.

> Nudity is still illegal in most American states.

Chlamydia

Virtually unheard of just a few years ago, chlamydia is now reputed to be the commonest sexually transmitted disease in the western world. It is a common cause of problems among new born babies and causes sterility in thousands of women every year. It is also believed to be the cause of approximately fifty per cent of all cases of female pelvic inflammatory disease.

The importance of chlamydia only became apparent when researchers into the condition known as Non Specific Urethritis (also known as NSU and Non Gonococcal Urethritis) found that in about half the cases the organism responsible was chlamydia. Non Specific Genital Infection is also likely to be caused by chlamydia.

The symptoms of chlamydia mean that it is often mistaken for gonorrhoea. Women who have the disease may have pain on passing urine and a vaginal discharge. Men get similar symptoms – burning on passing urine and a discharge.

The difference between chlamydia and gonorrhoea is that when penicillin is given chlamydia infections do not clear up. Other drugs such as tetracycline or erythromycin are needed to control chlamydia.

Circumcision (female)

Female circumcision is brutal, unnecessary and barbaric and usually involves the removal of all or part of the clitoris and sensitive areas around it. It is done to prevent a woman enjoying sex. The theory behind it is that a circumcised woman will be less likely to be unfaithful to her husband since she will get relatively little pleasure from sex.

> Having sex – or even thinking about it – makes a man's hair grow faster.

CIRCUMCISION (MALE)

Circumcision of the male is sometimes essential. When the foreskin really cannot be pulled back properly it may need to be removed. But this operation is performed far more often than is necessary. Performing the operation for social, religious or cosmetic purposes is as brutal and inexcusable as circumcision of the female.

By desensitising the normally sensitive parts of the penis (e.g. the glans) circumcision may affect a man's ability to enjoy sexual intercourse.

CLITORIS

The clitoris contains the same sort of erectile tissue as is in the penis, and like the penis the clitoris fills with blood and swells during sexual excitement. Like the penis, again, it has a small covering – rather like a foreskin. The size and shape of the clitoris varies a great deal from one woman to another but when unstimulated the clitoris is usually no bigger than a pea. It contains numerous nerve endings and is exquisitely tender to the touch. The clitoris is one of the most powerful, most responsive and most influential organs in the female body. Its sole function seems to be to provide sexual pleasure.

In some women the clitoris is stimulated quite naturally during ordinary intercourse since as the labia minora are pulled and pushed by the penis moving in and out of the vagina so the clitoris is gently massaged by the movement. Sometimes, however, the movement of the labial hood over the clitoris is not enough to produce an adequate sexual response and the clitoris may need to be stimulated directly – usually by the finger tips – although the clitoris is so sensitive that this has to be done carefully. When stimulated properly the clitoris gets bigger and much harder.

> In the UK the penalty for having sex with a live cod is life imprisonment. But you can have sex with a dead cod with no worries.

Coitus Interruptus

The theory is that if he takes his penis out of her vagina before he ejaculates then she won't get pregnant. This very old fashioned method costs nothing and is widely used but isn't very efficient. Just before ejaculation a few drops of liquid usually leak out from the end of the penis – and these drops may contain some sperm. Many pregnancies among women over the age of forty result from the use of this method because she is too old to take the pill and too embarrassed to buy a packet of condoms and both she and her partner imagines that she is too old to get pregnant.

Conception

A woman can only have a baby when a male sperm meets a female egg.

Eggs which are produced by the ovaries, get into the uterus by travelling along one of the two Fallopian tubes. The ovaries are the female equivalent of the male testicles; they manufacture the female sex hormones oestrogen and progesterone and they store a supply of approximately half a million immature eggs.

Roughly once every twenty eight days an egg will mature and leave the ovary ready for conception. Less than one in a thousand eggs will ever reach the uterus. The rest are 'spares'.

If sperm manage to get up the vagina, through the cervix and into the uterus at roughly the same time as an egg is released and available then the sperm may fertilise the egg. If this happens then a baby will start to grow.

If there are no sperm handy when the egg is waiting then the endometrium (the special lining that the uterus develops every month in case a foetus needs supporting) won't be needed and can be discharged as a monthly bleed. Then the whole cycle begins again.

> In China busy men used to deal with business matters while making love to their mistresses. They would sign papers and do deals while still physically connected to their lovers.

Condoms

Also known as the sheath, the condom is the only mass market contraceptive designed for use by men.

The condom is probably the most widely used contraceptive in the world today — with over 100,000,000 people using them regularly. You can buy condoms that are straight or contoured, transparent or coloured, thin or very thin, smooth or ribbed. You can buy them with or without a lubricant. You can buy them with or without a teat on the end to catch the sperm. Well made condoms stretch and are pretty tough. (They can, however, be torn by teeth or nails.) Condoms are useful for unplanned moments, they are convenient, they can be bought by either sex, they are readily available in most parts of the world, they produce very few side effects, they can help to delay orgasm if he suffers from premature ejaculation, they are cheap and they provide good protection against sexually transmitted diseases. A condom will only work properly if used properly. It should be put onto the penis as soon as the penis becomes erect (some couples make this part of their foreplay — she 'dresses' his penis as soon as possible) and removed after ejaculation and before the penis goes limp again. Artificial lubricants should not be used since they may weaken the material. If she has particularly powerful vaginal muscles she should be careful (particularly in the 'woman on top' positions) since she may succeed in 'sucking' the condom off his penis. When the condom fails to provide protection it is usually because of over eagerness or carelessness.

Contraception

Egyptian women were mixing honey and crocodile dung into contraceptive pessaries four thousand years ago. Arabian women made contraceptives from pomegranate pulps treated with alum and rocksalt, and the Greek author Aristotle described a chemical con-

> There are ninety different positions in which a man and a woman can have sex.

coction, consisting of cedar oil, frankincense and olive oil. During the sixteenth century Japanese men wore sheaths made of tortoiseshell, horn or leather. European men wore sheaths made of moistened linen. Chinese women used to cover the entrances to their wombs with discs of oiled tissue paper. In Persia women who didn't want to get pregnant were advised to take nine backward jumps after sex. Coitus interruptus – in which the male partner withdraws just before he ejaculates – was widely practised by the Hebrews and is probably the oldest known form of birth control.

see also: Cervical cap, Coitus Interruptus, Condom, Contraceptive Pill, Diaphragm, Intra Uterine Contraceptive Device (IUCD), Morning After Pills, Rhythm Method, Spermicidal Creams, Sterilisation

Contraceptive Pill

There are scores of different brands of contraceptive pill. In view of the ever changing variety of products available you should visit your doctor or family planning clinic for advice.

Cystitis

Cystitis – an inflammation of the bladder – is particularly common among women because the female urethra (the tube that carries urine down from the bladder) is much shorter and more vulnerable to infection than the male urethra.

The two symptoms most commonly associated with cystitis are: pain on passing urine and having to pass small amounts of urine unusually frequently. Other symptoms include the passing of cloudy, discoloured or blood stained urine.

There is a strong link between cystitis and sex, and 'honeymoon' cystitis is the name given to cystitis thought to have been

---

Prostitutes danced naked at the court of Pope Alexander VI. Prizes were then given to the men who had sex with the most women.

caused by sex. Brides are supposed to be exceptionally vulnerable to cystitis but 'honeymoon' cystitis is certainly not confined to brides.

Sex can cause bladder trouble in two ways.

First, if intercourse is particularly energetic the female urethra, which runs close to the vagina, may be subjected to a physical battering.

Second, an infection may be passed on during sex.

The problem can be minimised by:

- experimenting with different positions
- making sure that both partners wash thoroughly before sex
- avoiding aggressive thrusting or deep penetration
- emptying the bladder after sex to make sure that any bacteria around the entrance to the urethra are washed away
- placing a pillow under the woman's buttocks during sex in the missionary position
- making sure that the vagina is well lubricated before sex

Depression

Sex drive is linked closely to mood and a sudden or gradual loss of interest in sex may be associated with a feeling of depression.

There may be psychological causes for the depression (worry about specific problems such as work, children or money) or the depression may be caused by a physical problem (for example, the sort of hormone changes that can take place during or after childbirth or the menopause).

When there is a cause for a mood change then the solution is, of course, to deal with that underlying cause. Only then will interest in sex be restored.

> The Japanese people spend as much on buying sex as their government spends on education.

If you feel depressed for any reason then you should visit your doctor and ask for help, advice and treatment. (For advice on anxiety and depression see my book *How To Relax And Overcome Stress*.)

DIAPHRAGM

The diaphragm is a soft rubber disc fitted with a metal spring. Like the cap the diaphragm acts as a physical barrier – stopping the sperm from getting into the womb. It needs to be put into position before sex and left there until afterwards. Like the cap it provides no real protection against infection.

DISCOVERY (FEAR OF)

If you have no place where you can make love in comfort and private then your ability to enjoy sex will be severely affected by your fear of discovery. It is difficult to relax (an essential prerequisite to a successful orgasm) if you are worried about someone opening the living room door or shining a torch in through your car window or hearing the give away 'twang' of your bed springs. In such circumstances it is not unusual for sexual interest to decline altogether. The answer is usually to book an hour, a night or a weekend in a small hotel.

DISEASE (FEAR OF)

Similarly, neither partner will be able to relax if either one is worried about contracting a sexually transmitted disease.

DRUGS (EFFECT ON SEX LIFE)

If your interest in sex has disappeared or been reduced and/or your ability to enjoy sex has changed and you are taking a drug

---

Ejaculated sperm leaves the human penis faster than a sprinter leaves the blocks.

prescribed by your doctor or a drug that you have bought from the pharmacy then the chances are high that the drug you are taking is responsible for the changes in your sex life.

It is impossible to provide a full and up-to-date list of the drugs that can affect sexual interest and ability (the list changes constantly) but some of the types of drugs commonly associated with this problem include:

- tranquillisers
- sleeping tablets
- drugs for anxiety
- anti-depressants
- drugs used to control blood pressure
- drugs used to treat heart disease
- drugs used to treat headaches
- drugs used to treat fluid retention

This list is not by any means comprehensive.

If you think that your sex life could have been affected by drugs that have been prescribed by your doctor or that you have bought from a pharmacy then you should consult your doctor or pharmacist straight away.

Do NOT stop the suspected drug until you have spoken to your doctor or pharmacist because this may cause additional problems – and if you need to stop the drug you may need to do so slowly.

If the drug you are taking could be responsible there may be an alternative that you can try that does not produce this side effect.

ERECTION

In some animals the male penis develops an erection automatically whenever a female approaches – as long as she is in heat. But male

> The average quantity of sperm produced in a single ejaculation is 5mls – a teaspoonful. But the world record is 31cc – two soup spoonfuls.

humans don't automatically acquire an erection every time a female gets close and it is not necessary for the female to be 'in heat' for a male to acquire an erection.

The reflex action mechanism which enables a human penis to become erect functions more or less from birth and it is common for babies who are no more than a day or so old to have erections as a result of an automatic erectile reflex – though it is not known how the reflex is triggered or what does the triggering.

Just before puberty the ability of the penis to become erect increases dramatically and it is perfectly possible for boys of nine or ten years of age to have serviceable erections.

In most adult men the development of an erection is not under voluntary control – it either comes or it doesn't. The exceptions are those yogi who have enough control over their bodies to produce erections by deliberate thought processes. Sexual stimulation is the usual reason for the development of an erection and regular activity improves the efficiency of the reflex. A man who has sex often will find it easier to have an erection than a man who has sex only rarely. Impotence can develop through disuse.

(Although the erection reflex is normally triggered only by sexual stimuli it can be triggered by non sexual stimuli in the right circumstances. A French sex expert reported the case of a man who had sex a number of times in a room lit by a green light. Eventually the man automatically had an erection whenever he saw a green light. I rather suspect that this must have made city driving a hazardous if stimulating adventure.)

Normally, when a penis is limp the numerous arteries inside the organ are kept closed and empty of blood by tightened muscles in the penis. At the start of an erection the muscle fibres inside the penis become relaxed and loose allowing blood to flow into the arteries and to fill the spongy tissues of the penis. The flow of blood into the penis compresses the veins which normally carry blood

---

A Frenchman who is 6 foot 8 inches tall has a wife who is 4 foot 11 inches small. They cannot kiss and make love at the same time.

away from the penis with the result that the penis rapidly gets larger. The penis rises into an upright position as it becomes firm because there is more of the spongy, erectile tissue on its lower side and when this tissue fills with blood and expands it forces the whole penis upwards and into a shape and form better suited for sliding into the vagina.

It was at one time thought that a penis was either erect or non erect but research has shown that the erectile state of a penis is constantly changing. It has been said that erections are to the penis what earthquakes are to the earth, in that although large earthquakes are clearly noticeable the earth does have small, hardly noticed earthquakes all the time.

The circumstances which help to create an erection are easily influenced by other factors – noticeably psychological ones such as fear, hope and embarrassment. On some occasions the penis will become erect against the will of, and to the embarrassment of, its owner whereas on other occasions the penis will ignore attempts to encourage a response and will steadfastly refuse to become erect whatever entreaties may be made (and whoever makes them).

Once an erection develops it will usually last no more than two or three minutes. (This may not sound very long but it is a lifetime compared to some animals. An elephant's erection lasts around thirty seconds while a chimpanzee's partner can expect a delay of only about ten seconds between the onset of an erection and ejaculation. On the other hand the human male is a sexual incompetent when compared to the male ferret who is likely to have an erection lasting up to eight hours. The dog's penis seems to stay erect for longer than it really does because after penetration and ejaculation it swells at the base and therefore deflates very slowly – allowing the male to keep his penis inside the female for much longer than would otherwise be possible.)

Most men have their greatest number of erections in their

One in five women perform oral sex because they enjoy it – the rest do it because their partners enjoy it.

late teens and early twenties. Erections and nocturnal emissions of semen during erotic dreams (wet dreams) are an inevitable part of growing up for a boy, and teenage boys have sexuality thrust upon them whether they are ready for it or not.

Older men have a much greater chance of having a good erection in the morning rather than at night. There are three reasons for this: firstly, a full bladder is common early in the morning and a full bladder helps to produce a stronger erection; secondly, erotic dreams are more common in the early morning than late at night and thirdly, a good night's rest helps to give the older male a chance to build up his strength.

Erogenous Zones

Touching is very therapeutic – and yet most of us do it far too infrequently.

When small children are not regularly shown love they quickly become depressed and stop eating. A child who isn't cuddled can die of love starvation as truly as a child who isn't fed can die of food starvation. Children who are deprived of cuddles and love when they are small often grow up with deep rooted psychological and emotional problems. They may become promiscuous in their constant, never-to-be-satisfied search for love.

Researchers all around the world have shown that it isn't just children who benefit from kissing and cuddling. Insurance companies in America have found that if a wife kisses her husband goodbye when he goes off to work every morning he will be less likely to have a car accident on the way to the office or the factory. He will, on average, live five years longer than if she doesn't give him a morning kiss. Without physical signs of affection we become more brittle, less emotionally stable and more susceptible to fear, pressure and distress.

> One in three men has had a condom break during sex and hasn't told his partner.

~ Sex ~

Of course, touching isn't just reassuring.

The right sort of touch, at the right time, in the right place, can be extremely arousing and stimulating.

Some people imagine that the only place to touch one another during foreplay is below the belt. But that is not true.

The average human body is covered with approximately two square metres of skin. Some of that skin contains areas of special sexual sensitivity — the genital areas and the lips are clearly erogenous — but any piece of skin on your body can become an erogenous zone if it is stimulated in the right way. The skin is a massive — and extremely complex — organ of sexual response and sexual communication. Some women (and some men) can reach the heights of sexual excitement if a lover blows onto their skin or if their arms are stroked or if their backs are massaged very gently with the finger tips. At different times and in different circumstances both men and women will appreciate being touched, held, licked, nibbled, pinched (gently), slapped (gently) and stroked.

The trick, of course, is knowing where you can find the really erogenous zones. If you know where your partner's erogenous zones are then you can turn him or her on like a light!

To begin with try dragging your fingernails gently across the skin. Move your fingers slowly and then quickly, in circles and spirals. Stroke and massage along every erogenous zone. Touch the stomach, the thighs, the backs of the knees and around the navel. Scratch the palms of both hands lightly with your nails. Blow in his or her ear. And then try blowing gently on his or her spine. Kiss and then lick the most responsive spots and then blow on them while they are still wet. Penetrate her or his body symbolically by moving your finger rhythmically into and out of his navel, ear or mouth.

Learn to kiss properly.

Relax your mouth, let your lips go limp. Then kiss everywhere that you have touched.

> Men consider a nice bottom just as important as intelligence when trying to find an ideal woman.

Practise on the palm of your hand to see the difference between a hard, clenched kiss and a soft, limp, thoroughly relaxed kiss. Brush your partner's skin with your lips. Drag your lips along their most erogenous zones.

Men tend to be very sensitive:
- on and around their nipples
- in and around their navels
- in their armpits
- inside their upper thighs
- at the nape of their necks
- along the length of their spines
- on the inside of their elbows
- behind their knees
- on their buttocks
- on their throats
- around their ears

You may find that some areas are too sensitive for you to touch for long. Once you have worked your way around his body then you can move in on the predictably erogenous bits.

For most men the most sensitive part is usually the frenulum – the small piece of skin on the underside of the penis, where the glans meets the shaft. Next, comes the tip of the penis, the edge of the glans, the shaft and the testicles.

Men are usually very sensitive in the area between their genitalia and their anus and are also very likely to be sensitive to touch in and around the anus.

If you are shy about touching his sexual organs say so. Try touching very gently for just a second or two at a time. Be as cautious as you like. You will soon see the extraordinary amount of pleasure you can give with your fingertips. Don't rush yourself. Progress day by day.

Women tend to be very sensitive:

Up to one in seven cases of chronic impotence are caused by penile injuries sustained during masturbation or intercourse.

- on and around their nipples
- in and around their navels
- in their armpits
- inside their upper thighs
- at the nape of their necks
- along the length of their spines
- on the inside of their elbows
- behind their knees
- on their buttocks
- on their throats
- around their ears

Some areas may be too sensitive for you to touch for long. A few women find that their nipples are too sensitive to fondled.

Once you have worked your way around her body then you can move in on the predictably erogenous bits. For women the clitoris is usually the most sensitive of all sensitive parts, followed by the inner lips of the vagina and then the outer lips. Some women say that one part of their vagina may be more sensitive than any other.

Women are usually very sensitive in the area between their genitalia and their anus and are also very likely to be sensitive to touch in and around the anus.

If you are shy about touching her sexual organs say so. Try touching very gently for just a second or two at a time. Be as cautious as you like. You will soon see the extraordinary amount of pleasure you can give with your fingertips. Don't rush yourself. Progress day by day.

Exhaustion

Stress, anxiety and overwork are all enemies of sex. Any man or woman who is under too much pressure will, inevitably, find that his or her interest in sex will fall away rapidly.

Nine out of ten penises are between 5 and 7 inches long when fully erect.

Tiredness and exhaustion mean that going to bed is a chance to rest or to sleep – rather than an opportunity to experiment with new sexual positions.

This problem affects millions of men and women whose daily commitments are so great that sex is gradually pushed to one side. The more determined, the more ambitious and the more hard working an individual is the greater the chance that his or her sex life will be pushed to one side. The more caring, the more compassionate and the more thoughtful an individual is the greater the chance that sex will take second, third or even fourth place in his or her life.

Men and women with careers and men and women who look after the home and the children all suffer from this problem. Even if they can find the time or the enthusiasm for sex they can't find the energy.

If your sex life has been crushed by your other interests – and it worries you – then the only way to deal with the problem is to sort out your priorities and to allocate your time more carefully.

Fantasies

Sexual fantasies don't mean anything. They are created out of hopes, guilts, longings, prejudices, fears and hidden desires. In our fantasies we can enjoy raw mind sex and explore every dark recess of lust without inhibition or recrimination. There is no need for caution or condoms in fantasy land. Your mind is a virtual reality machine which can turn wishful thinking into erotic playland. There are no limits, no restrictions, no conventions and no hidden agendas. Fantasy sex is the ultimate in safe sex. The bizarre world in which you venture during fantasy time bears no relationship to real life.

Don't try to analyse your fantasies: just enjoy them. And don't worry about them: fantasies say nothing about how you would wish to behave in real life.

Three out of four women say that their sexual pleasure is not affected by penis size.

~ Sex ~

What sort of things do men fantasise about?

When adolescent boys start fantasizing their dreams are largely physical. They fantasise about seducing beautiful women – often mothers of their friends or friends of their mother. They fantasise about physical sex. As they grow older their fantasies become more complicated. Here are the most popular male sexual fantasies:

1. Replacing their usual partner with another woman (friend, neighbour, young girl, film star, past lover).
2. Having sex with a woman who resists but finds it so exciting that she gives in.
3. Watching other people have sex.
4. Watching another man (or several men) have sex with their partner.
5. Having group sex.
6. Having a homosexual encounter.
7. Being sexually abused by women. One man reported that his favourite sexual fantasy was to be tied to a conveyor belt and carried past a line of beautiful women. Each time the belt came to a new woman she would climb on top of him. When she'd finished the conveyor belt would take him on to the next woman.
8. Having sex in public while an audience watches.
9. Making love in bizarre circumstances.
10. Taking part in a threesome with a man and a woman or two women.
11. Forcing a woman to have sex with an animal.
12. Watching two women have sex together.
13. Watching a regular partner work as a prostitute.
14. Being raped by a woman.
15. Being spanked.
16. Being involved in food fights with a woman.

> A woman in the north of England claims that by massaging semen onto her breasts every day for nine years she increased their size from 34B to 34D.

17. Being urinated on by a woman.
18. Being a slave to a woman.
19. Being subjected to anal sex by a woman equipped with a large dildo.
20. Having sex with a woman with huge breasts.

What sort of things do women fantasise about?

Girls' fantasies begin by being more emotional than physical. Young girls fantasise about being loved.

But in adult life women's fantasies become more physical and are often just as explicit as male fantasies. Here are some of the most popular female fantasies.

1. Being raped.
2. Being forced to have sex in public.
3. Being exposed in public.
4. Having sex with a lover in a public place.
5. Making love to young boys.
6. Making love to an animal.
7. Being sexually abused by several men at once.
8. Being taken by a stranger from behind – never seeing his face.
9. Watching others have sex.
10. Having an encounter with a stranger who leaves after sex.
11. Having a lesbian encounter.
12. Stripping on stage.
13. Taking part in a group sexual encounter.
14. Working as a prostitute.
15. Humiliating a man.
16. Being tied down and used by a series of men.
17. Being spanked.
18. Having a male slave.
19. Being forced to perform oral sex on a man.

In old Jewish law the punishment for anyone caught masturbating was execution.

~ Sex ~

20. Taking part in a threesome with two men or one man and a woman.

Do fantasies ever turn into reality?

Sometimes. But not very often. A fantasy is not necessarily a repressed wish. Women commonly fantasise about being taken forcibly or raped by several men at once. For them the fantasy is entirely different to reality. Similarly, men who fantasise about raping women should not feel guilty; the fantasy is a long way from the real thing.

Foreplay

One of the things most women regularly complain about is their partner's reluctance – or refusal – to spend much time on foreplay.

'I get really fed up,' complained one woman, 'when my husband comes up behind me when I'm doing the washing up and instantly wants to make love to me – whether I'm in the mood for it or not.'

'Nothing annoys me more,' said another, 'than getting into bed and suddenly finding him lying on top of me without a word of warning or the remotest attempt at seduction.'

It is usually men who are guilty of over eagerness and a lack of understanding. But it isn't only men. Some women are as guilty as the worst men – always wrongly assuming that men are for ever ready for action.

For both sexes foreplay is usually just as important as sex itself. (Though there are exceptions, of course. Occasionally, a couple will want to plunge straight into steamy sex without any preliminaries. But this is usually either because the flirtation has been so successful that both partners are ready for sex or because the two partners have been separated for a long time. When this hap-

---

In 1300 BC, when King Menephta returned home to Egypt after defeating the Libyans, he took with him 13,000 penises which he had cut from 13,000 enemies.

pens buttons will fly and material will rip and foreplay will seem entirely unnecessary.) Most people need to get into the mood to enjoy sex. And that means more than just a few moments of crude fondling. It means thought, care and tenderness.

Gonorrhoea

Still one of the commonest sexually transmitted diseases. Of all the women who contract gonorrhoea sixty per cent will have no symptoms at all. The rest will usually notice fairly vague, non specific symptoms such as a vaginal discharge and a burning on passing urine (the same symptoms as are found with chlamydia). The symptoms of gonorrhoea usually develop within two to ten days of having sex with an infected partner.

Diagnosing and treating gonorrhoea is important because the disease can cause pelvic infections and sterility in women. In addition if a woman with gonorrhoea gives birth her baby can contract an extremely unpleasant eye infection.

G Spot

Although the clitoris is universally acknowledged as the source of sexual satisfaction in women some researchers claim that there is also a small bean shaped patch of erectile tissue attached to the inside of the top part of the vagina and situated 2.5 to 5 cms inside it. This area – known as the G spot – is said to be directly behind the pubic bone and is claimed to be 2.5 to 4 cms across. It is known as the G spot after its discoverer; Ernst Grafenberg, a German gynaecologist.

Grafenberg found the G spot during the 1940s when he was researching different methods of birth control. His claim that when stimulated by pressure the G spot triggers a vaginal orgasm substantiated previous, controversial claims that women can have two

> One in ten women have never had an orgasm.

different types of orgasm – one sort triggered by stimulation of the clitoris and the other triggered by movement inside the vagina.

In addition to producing an orgasm, stimulation of the G spot is also alleged to produce a fluid. Three American researchers have claimed that the G spot is a sort of female prostate gland. It has been argued that the spot (or patch of tissue or gland) secretes a special fluid during orgasm and that women do, therefore, ejaculate when they reach a climax.

Despite all these claims there is still a considerable amount of controversy among gynaecologists about whether or not the G spot really does exist and whether or not it has any sexually active function.

Gynaecologists are rather wary about looking for it since they fear that if they find it their patients may get the wrong idea.

Pathologists report that they are unable to find the patch when dissecting dead bodies but those who believe in its existence argue that this is because the G spot atrophies with age.

Some experts, finding the existence of the G spot difficult to substantiate in the absence of any hard evidence, claim that the spot only exists in some women and that only a few women ejaculate.

There are a large number of gynaecologists and sex experts who do not believe in the existence of a G spot at all.

HERPES

Herpes is not a new disease. The Roman emperor Tiberius tried to stamp it out by banning kissing, and Shakespeare wrote about it in Romeo and Juliet.

There are two types of herpes – herpes simplex 1 (HSV1) and herpes simplex 2 (HSV2) – but there are many different strains of the viruses. Both types of virus can infect either the mouth or the genital area and although herpes can be transmitted sexually it can also be transmitted in other ways. It is possible to get herpes

> Nine out of ten teenage boys fantasise sexually during masturbation. (What the hell do the rest think about? Homework?)

more than once – because of the existence of different types of virus.

The first symptoms of a herpes infection can appear up to thirty years after the virus first arrived on the skin – an infected mother washing her child can give it herpes which does not erupt until half a lifetime later. The herpes HSV2 can live for seventy two hours on towels, clothing and lavatory seats.

Although it does not get as much publicity as it used to get herpes is still increasing very rapidly. Ironically, the increase is at least partly due to improving social conditions. A generation or two ago most people acquired immunity to herpes when they were exposed to the infection as children, but these days we rarely share baths or towels with one another and so we grow up without ever being exposed to the herpes viruses. As a result we do not develop any immunity to them and are far more vulnerable when we reach adulthood.

Babies are very much at risk. Herpes is said to kill about one baby in every 250,000 in the western world – with half of those babies acquiring the infection from their mothers and the other half from visitors or nurses. If a pregnant woman has active herpes the danger can be minimised by delivering her baby by Caesarian section.

The first symptoms of herpes usually appear gradually. A few days, perhaps a week after sexual contact with someone carrying the infection, the sufferer will feel a little tired. He may have a fever and a headache and may also suffer from stiffness and backache.

As these general symptoms develop so more specific symptoms will appear. There will be some local genital irritation and very probably a discharge. There may also be pain or burning when urine is passed. About four days after the onset of the irritation small blisters will probably appear on the penis (or around the va-

---

Nine out of ten men lose their virginity before their 19th birthday.

gina in the case of a woman) and these may well be extremely sore. The glands in the groin will usually swell too.

Severe recurrences of herpes are relatively rare and around a third of sufferers have just one attack and no more. Another third of sufferers get occasional, infrequent and relatively minor outbreaks. Only a third of herpes sufferers get troublesome recurrences – and those are usually less painful than the initial attacks.

Things to remember about herpes:
1. Avoid having sex when a herpes lesion is visible.
2. Wash your hands carefully after visiting the toilet.
3. Don't sit on the seats in public lavatories.
4. Be gentle during sex if you have herpes – trauma can bring back symptoms.
5. Use plenty of lubrication during sex to keep friction to a minimum.
6. A condom will provide some protection – as will barrier creams.
7. Don't kiss or touch cold sores or genital sores.
8. Remember that stress and anxiety can make herpes lesions worse.

IMPOTENCE

Impotence always seems to be the end of the world to a previously virile male. It usually strikes at the most inopportune and most embarrassing moment. It certainly strikes at a moment when a man is most vulnerable.

The symptoms are simple: he cannot acquire an erection easily and/or if he does get one then it is either too feeble or too short lived to enable him to penetrate his partner.

Here are some of the most likely causes of impotence. (Incidentally, age does not really figure on the list of possible causes. Age can affect the amount of time a man must wait for his second erection but it is not itself a cause of impotence.)

> A man whose penis got stuck in the cold tap in his bath claimed that he had been using his unfortunate organ to try and clear a blockage.

Alcohol
A modest amount of alcohol will increase the desire for sex but too much will adversely affect performance. Most 'leisure' drugs can cause problems. Smoking is also a major cause of impotence.

Anxiety
Anxiety about failure is a common cause of impotence. The risk of failure is proportional to the build up. If a man really wants to impress his partner then the chances of his being impotent are high. Men who worry about how well they are doing are also prone to impotence. A man who is making love to a woman he really loves (or fancies) for the first time will often discover that he is impotent; his desire to do well will be too much for him.

Disease
Diseases such as diabetes can cause impotence.

Drugs
Prescribed drugs – particularly drugs which are used in the treatment of high blood pressure or depression.

Fear
Many types of fear can produce impotence. A man will have difficulty in acquiring an erection if he is frightened of catching a disease, of being caught, of making his partner pregnant, of hurting her or causing himself pain.

Guilt
A married man who tries to make love to a woman other than his wife will be prone to impotence.

Six out of ten people prefer to have sex with the lights off.

~ Sex ~

Inadequacy
Some men feel very inadequate about their bodies, not simply about the size or shape of their penises. Some men cannot comfortably make love to women whom they consider to be beautiful – they may feel happier with a woman who is very plain, who takes no pride in herself or even a woman who is deformed. Blind prostitutes, prostitutes with amputated limbs and prostitutes with severe, disabling disorders often do surprisingly well.

Memories
Memories can cause problems. A man who tries to make love in a room or bed he associates with someone else may suffer from impotence, as may a man who tries to make love to a woman who has been a friend or a former partner of a friend for many years.

Obesity
Men who are fat are more likely to suffer from impotence. (Sexual positions in which the woman is on top are most suitable for men who are severely overweight).

Tiredness
Tiredness, often through overwork, is a common cause of impotence and it is quite normal to have difficulty in acquiring or maintaining an erection when tired.

Here are some tips for the man suffering from impotence.

1. The first and most important thing to remember is that impotence probably affects every man in the world at one time or another. If you do occasionally get an erection (asleep or awake, alone or with a partner) then there is probably nothing wrong with your equipment. The problem is likely to be in your mind

---

An Arab holds the world record for the longest lasting erection – 60 days.

---

and can be conquered. The vast majority of cases of impotence fit into this category.
2. The more you worry about the problem the worse it will get.
3. If you are totally unable to have an erection at any time then your problem may need treatment with hormones. Talk to your doctor.
4. Do not waste your money on 'quack' remedies. Back in the eighteenth century in Italy impotent men presented their sluggish and reluctant organs to St. Damien and begged for help. Today men are more likely to pay for weird concoctions. Because of the shame and embarrassment that they feel, impotent men often visit 'quack' healers secretly and dare not complain when the product turns out to be worthless.
5. If you are suffering from impotence you must slowly and gradually rebuild your confidence. You should try to deal with any anxieties or problems in other parts of your life and you should spend a little time learning how to relax. You will find it easier to conquer your impotence if you have a regular partner rather than a number of occasional partners or a succession of one night stands.

   With new partners you will have to explain your problem repeatedly and will undoubtedly find it more stressful.
6. Spend time on foreplay. Learn how to please your partner in ways other than full intercourse. If you know that you can bring your partner to orgasm before you have entered her then the pressure on you will be reduced enormously. Try to relax with your partner as often as you can – and to cuddle and kiss frequently.
7. Some experts recommend that if you are suffering from impotence you should make a decision to try not to have sex for six weeks. During that time, they say, you should concentrate on touching your partner. You should become adept at foreplay.

> If rice crops are in danger of failing, villagers in Java are expected to have sex as often as they can to help ensure the fertility of the crops.

~ Sex ~

Even if you have an erection you should not have sex. You should learn to relax and enjoy your partner. Bring her to orgasm with your hands and encourage her to do the same for you.

If, after six weeks, you are regularly getting erections then you can make love. If not then you should extend your period of deliberate abstinence for another four weeks. Taking the pressure off in this way can work wonders.

8. Finally, if your erection is a poor one you will find that penetration is far easier to achieve if you lie side by side or if your partner sits on top of you. The missionary position is not good for men who suffer from partial impotence.

INADEQUACY (FEAR OF)

Thousands of perfectly sensible, perfectly good looking and otherwise sane and confident individuals suffer agonies because of fears that their bodies or their sexual skills are inadequate.

The first part of the problem is undoubtedly inspired by the photographs of abnormal women (and occasionally men) in magazines and newspapers. Female models who pose professionally for the camera are usually either boyishly thin (if they are being hired to sell dresses) or absurdly and abnormally voluptuous (if they are being hired to grace the pages of men's magazines). It is not surprising that looking at these photographs gives many women an inferiority complex. When men are photographed or filmed naked they are often equipped with sexual equipment of heroic proportions.

The second part of the problem is inspired partly by those commentators and journalists who write so glibly and easily about the (imaginary) sex lives of the rich and famous (and who succeed in making most ordinary people feel woefully inadequate), partly by the 'experts' who, when they write about sexual matters usually do so with a startling confidence and an unerring ability to raise

---

> Surgeons in Japan regularly turn sexually experienced women back into virgins by fitting them with new hymens.

expectations, offering their readers hopes and aspirations that are incompatible with reality, and partly by novelists who write about sex in a way that is quite divorced from reality.

Women who fail to achieve multiple orgasms every time they have sex are encouraged to believe that there must be something wrong either with them or with their partners, and men who cannot sustain an erection for long enough for their partners to achieve orgasm mistakenly believe that they are sexually incompetent.

Unrealistic expectations produce anxiety and inadequacy.

Men expect women to be sultry and bubbling with passion and regularly to experience orgasms which leave them sobbing, exhausted and drained.

Women expect men to have organs two foot long, to have the power and the strength of a lion and to make love for hours on end. In the real world he may complain of backache, and she may (genuinely) have a migraine and the noisy bedsprings may wake the children.

The wit and the romance and the fun have, to a large extent, been removed from sex and replaced by standards, rights and expectations.

We may be more enlightened and less prudish than our ancestors but we have created our own range of social and sexual stresses. We have been encouraged to accept the 'abnormal' as the 'normal' and as a result dissatisfaction, frustration and unhappiness are rife.

Guilt, self doubt and inadequacy produce either frigidity or impotence or a total disinterest and disinclination to take any interest in sex. Millions are crippled by the fear of failure. No one points out that sex is just one small part of an understanding and enjoyable relationship.

> Couples who live together but aren't married have sex three times as often as couples who live together and are married.

~ Sex ~

Intra Uterine Contraceptive Device

The IUCD consists of a small piece of curved plastic or metal which is put into the womb to stop a baby developing. Many women find them to be safe, effective, comfortable and convenient. They can be left in place for months at a time and are not usually displaced by tampons, bleeding or sex. They do not interfere with sexual pleasure and it is fairly easy to check that they are still in place by feeling for the thread which should poke out through the cervix.

Occasionally, the IUCD can cause heavy bleeding, a vaginal discharge and cramp like pains and rarely an IUCD may work its way through the wall of the womb and into the abdomen.

There are some stories of babies being born triumphantly holding their mother's IUCD in their tiny hands.

Light (on or off?)

Some people hate doing it with the light on. Some find it difficult to get aroused with the light off.

Women – or men – who are shy about making love with the light on are usually either worried about their own bodies or worried about what they'll see. Some married men and women have never seen their partner naked.

The answer may be to find a suitable compromise.

If you have opposing fancies put a low intensity bulb into a bedside lamp and fit it with a heavy (but safe and suitable) shade (don't drape an article of clothing over it or else you may be interrupted by the smell of burning).

Or keep the lights on but make love under the duvet.

The shy one among you may then be able to get accustomed to nudity bit by bit.

In the 18th century the London Stock Exchange kept its own brothel.

Loss of Interest In Sex

When men and women are asked to list the things that worry them most about sex they frequently put 'lack of interest' very near to the top.

What many people fail to understand is that it is normal to have a decreasing interest in sex as the years go by – particularly if you share your life with one partner.

When a relationship begins sex is often extremely important. Newly weds frequently make love many times a week – often, many times a day. But as the weeks and months go by it is normal for that initial enthusiasm to fade. Gradually, other aspects of the relationship become increasingly important. Friendship and companionship grow in significance. And after a year or two most married couples will privately admit that a regular sex life is less important than having someone to love, care for and share things with. Gradually, other things become more important. Work, family, hobbies and friends all start to take precedence over sex.

Unfortunately, when people are asked about how often they make love they invariably lie. People don't like admitting that they make love once a month (or even less often) and so when questioned they say that they still make love two or three times a week.

Such white lies help to keep the myth (and the guilt) going. When the next lot of interviewees are asked how often they have sex they lie too. No one wants to admit that their sex life is less than 'normal'. What they do not realise is that there is a great difference between what they think is 'normal' and what really is 'normal'.

There is a story about American President Coolidge which illustrates this phenomenon extremely well.

Coolidge was visiting an American farm with his wife and soon after their arrival the President and his wife were taken off on separate tours. When Mrs Coolidge passed the chicken pens she asked the keeper how often the rooster made love to his hens.

The average woman takes 4.5 minutes to masturbate to orgasm.

~ Sex ~

'Dozens of times,' answered the keeper, undoubtedly rather surprised and probably a little embarrassed.

'Please tell that to the President,' said Mrs Coolidge with a sly smile.

When Mr Coolidge's half of the tour arrived at the chicken house the keeper passed on the information.

'Same hen every time?' asked the President.

'Oh, no, Mr President!' answered the keeper. 'A different one each time.'

Mr Coolidge nodded wisely. 'Please tell that to Mrs Coolidge,' he instructed the keeper.

The slowing down in the frequency of love making is not peculiar to the human species. It happens in other species too, and like humans it is often only the introduction of a new partner which triggers an increase in sexual activity.

At the start of any physical relationship most couples try different techniques to keep their sex life alive. But the possibilities are, in reality, limited and are often exhausted after a few months. What was once exciting becomes routine and other things assume greater importance. Eventually, in most relationships, a comfortable pattern develops. If the relationship is a good one then sex will eventually play just a small part in keeping the couple together. Many relationships start off based on sex but end up being based on friendship.

There is nothing at all wrong with this change. It is perfectly normal.

But many people worry when they realise that they are not having sex as often as they were. They assume that there must be something wrong with the relationship. They worry that their partner does not find them attractive or does not love them. They feel inadequate. Often they look for things to blame.

If all the sparkle has gone from your relationship then you

In some parts of Africa all the wedding guests are expected to have sex with the bride. The bridegroom (literally) comes last.

may be able to put some of it back in. Flowers, candle-lit dinners, romantic weekends and lacy nightwear can put some thrills back into a well developed relationship. But the truth is that nothing can bring back that initial sense of physical excitement that heralds the start of a sexual relationship. You will never again rediscover that feeling of insatiability and you will never again have the feeling that you and your partner have invented sex.

Wise couples recognise that sexual habits and sexual patterns do change – in quality and quantity – with time. Sex may still be important and fun but it is no longer the sole reason for living and nor is it the glue that holds a relationship together.

Apart from a natural and inevitable (and, it has to be said, healthy and perfectly normal) lessening of interest in sex as a relationship blossoms there are many more specific (and more remediable) reasons why people lose their enthusiasm for sex.

See also: Celibacy, Depression, Discovery (Fear of), Disease (Fear of), Drug Therapy, Exhaustion, Inadequacy (Fear of), Pregnancy (Fear of), Repulsion

Masturbation

It used to be thought that masturbation was an exclusively male habit but it isn't. Women do it too. And no one need be afraid of long term consequences. No one ever went blind (or even short sighted) as a result of masturbating.

Masturbation is perfectly healthy, natural and normal. It isn't dirty and it isn't dangerous. It certainly isn't anything to be ashamed of. I doubt if there is anyone anywhere in the world who has never masturbated. Next time you see some pompous politician or industrialist on your TV screen remember that he or she will have almost certainly obtained pleasure through masturbation.

There are many times when it will be appropriate for one

A lesbian couple in Luxembourg have a collection of 186 different dildos.

partner to masturbate the other to an orgasm. If a woman has failed to orgasm during intercourse, for example, then her partner may help her to reach an orgasm by masturbating her.

Once again, this isn't anything to be ashamed about. Most women do not reach orgasm through sexual intercourse and need to masturbate (or to be masturbated) to reach satisfaction.

Many men and women feel shy or embarrassed about masturbation. Try not to allow your feelings to inhibit you. Talk to one another and show him (or her) what you would like him (or her) to do by moving his (or her) fingers a little in this direction and then a little in that direction. If you want him (or her) to press harder show him (or her) what you want.

When a man is masturbating a woman he should be slow and gentle. It is important not to just head straight for the clitoris. He should touch her general pubic area and the outer part of her vagina first. He should move his fingers up and down, round and round and from side to side. It's a good idea to start with a whole hand massage and to gradually concentrate on a smaller and smaller area (using fewer and fewer fingers) as he finds out what she wants. It is important to build up the speed and the pressure slowly.

He may find that she likes him to slip a finger in between her vaginal lips. Pressing the ball of the hand just above her pubic bone may be good for her. If she feels dry he may try dipping his (clean) fingers into her mouth and moistening her with saliva – as long as they are clean and healthy. If his hands are rough he should use baby oil or a plain hand cream. He should make sure that his fingernails are cut short and that there are no ragged edges. Gentle rubbing and pulling on the skin around the clitoris may produce just as good a result as touching the clitoris itself. With time a sensitive man will get to know what his partner wants but if he is in any doubt he should ask her to show him (with her fingers) what will give her most satisfaction.

If a man ejaculates twice a week he will have produced 500 ml of semen in a year.

When a woman is masturbating a man she may begin by gently dragging her nails along the skin of his scrotum and gently holding his scrotum in her fingers. She can try touching the skin underneath his scrotum and then gently running her fingers up and down the shaft of his penis.

She should hold his penis carefully between her fingers and move her fingers up and down. She should ask him if he wants her to hold him tighter – or not so tightly. If she needs a lubricant she can try saliva – as long as it is clean and healthy – or baby oil. She should speed up and slow down her movement to build up the suspense. If he has a foreskin she can move that upwards and downwards slowly. She can either grip his penis with her thumb and first finger or with the whole of her hand.

She should not be shy about watching when he ejaculates – he may find it an extra turn on. But do remember that when leaving the penis, semen may travel several feet.

Morning After Pill

Doctors can prescribe pills which prevent implantation should an egg have been fertilised. These pills need to be taken within hours of making love. The pills seem safe and effective. Doctors also sometimes use intrauterine contraceptive devices (IUCDs) as a form of post-sex contraception.

Oral Sex (Advice For Men)

Oral sex is a natural practice which millions regard as an enjoyable variation on other forms of sex – though naturally if either partner has or thinks he or she has any infection then oral sex should be avoided.

Oral sex involving a mouth and the female sexual organs is known as cunnilingus.

Some couples regularly have sex 1500 times a year – an average of 29 times a week.

~ Sex ~

The mouth is well designed for sex. The shape of the mouth, the lips and the tongue mean that stroking, kissing, licking, probing and penetrating are all possible. The mouth is well equipped with nerve endings, and taste buds enable the person performing oral sex to taste the juices which emerge from the vagina.

Many sex books discuss position 69 in which both partners perform oral sex on one another simultaneously. (To see where the position got its 'number' just look at the number.) The advantage of this twin position is that both partners are fully involved. But there are two main drawbacks. The first is that a partner who is approaching an orgasm may find it difficult to concentrate on what he or she is doing. The second drawback is that the position can be quite uncomfortable and difficult to get into.

It is usually easier to take turns at enjoying oral sex and it is usually better if the woman is on the receiving end first. Apart from sheer gallantry there are two simple reasons for this. First, women usually stay in the mood for sex after they have had an orgasm whereas men are prone to fall asleep. Second, a man will probably find that his erection develops while he is performing oral sex on his partner.

Although oral sex is very popular – and widely performed – some people are frightened of it.

If one partner is shy or hesitant then it is important that the other partner does not push things along too quickly. An introduction to oral sex can begin with a simple genital kiss, keeping the lips closed. Then, if both partners are willing and eager, progress can be made a little at a time on subsequent occasions.

It is usually thought that the person doing the sucking or kissing is adopting a passive or submissive role but in fact either partner can be dominant.

Women who want their partners to perform cunnilingus should make sure that they wash thoroughly beforehand. It is obvi-

---

According to an ancient Egyptian beauty tip a woman can improve the condition of her skin by bathing in a tub full of semen.

ously unreasonable to expect a partner to perform cunnilingus if there is any infection present.

And no man with an infection in or around his mouth or indeed in his body should perform cunnilingus either.

The clitoris is the most sensitive part of a woman's body. And it is extremely tender. Be careful with teeth and nails. It is often better to begin by kissing the labia minora and the entrance to the vagina. You can then run your tongue along and around the vaginal entrance. Stroking and kissing and touching will be more enjoyable for her than prodding, pushing or squeezing. You may like to try sliding your tongue into her vagina. Most men find the acid taste of vaginal juices pleasant and exciting. It is best to kiss around the clitoris rather than to kiss it directly.

Do not, repeat not, blow into the vagina. If you do then you may force air into the peritoneal cavity and that can be dangerous.

Here are three possible positions for cunnilingus

1. He lies on his back on the floor or bed. She gently lowers herself down onto him until her vagina meets his mouth. If she faces his feet she can use her hands to touch and caress his penis. If she is very flexible she may be able to lower herself forward to perform fellatio on him at the same time.

2. She sits on an ordinary chair. He kneels or squats in front of her. She wriggles to the front of the chair so that her vagina is exposed and close to his face.

3. She lies on her back with her knees drawn up towards her chest. He approaches her lying on his side. If her legs tire she can lower them so that her feet touch the floor on the other side of his head.

It is important to remember that a number of diseases can be transmitted via oral sex. Diseases can be transmitted from sexual organ to mouth or the other way. Unless you know that your part-

---

A couple in Sydney, Australia claims to have made love on 55 different Australian beaches.

ner is entirely free of disease you should not have any sort of sex with a partner without using some form of protection.

And if cunnilingus follows fellatio and kissing in the right order then – in theory at least – the result can be conception and, in nine months time, a baby. All that has to happen is that he comes in her mouth, she passes the semen to him in a kiss and he deposits the semen in her vagina from his mouth. Not impossible.

ORAL SEX (ADVICE FOR WOMEN)

Oral sex is a natural practice which millions regard as an enjoyable variation on other forms of sex – though naturally if either partner has an infection oral sex should be avoided.

Oral sex involving a mouth and the male sexual organs is known as fellatio.

The mouth is well designed for sex. The shape of the mouth, the lips and the tongue mean that stroking, kissing, licking, probing and penetrating are all possible. The mouth is well equipped with nerve endings and taste buds enable the person performing oral sex to taste the juices which emerge from the penis.

To perform fellatio you should begin by kissing the shaft and then the tip of his penis. The underside of the glans – particularly around the tip – is the most sensitive part. The testicles are also sensitive to the lips and tongue. Despite the fact that giving oral sex to a man is sometimes known as a 'blow job' it is important that you do NOT blow. Moisten his penis with the tongue and lick it as you would an ice cream. Then slip your lips around the glans of the penis and lower your head a little. Move your head up and down slowly and move your tongue around his penis.

There are of course many possible positions for fellatio – here are four:

1. He stands and she kneels in front of him.

Only 4% of women are virgins when they marry.

---

2. He sits in a chair. She kneels in front of him and lowers her head into his lap.
3. He lies flat on his back and she kneels over him.
4. He kneels on the floor and sits back on his haunches. She lies on the floor in front of him with her face in his lap.

When performing fellatio for the first time most women worry about the same thing: 'Will he come in my mouth?'

Ideally, this is something for couples to discuss together.

Whether or not he does come in her mouth is a question of taste – hers. And the same goes for whether or not she should spit or swallow. Some women like the salty, bitter taste of semen.

A reader of mine once told me that the most embarrassing moment of his life occurred when he went to dinner with his new girlfriend and her parents and had to listen for two and a half hours to his girlfriend and her mother discussing the advantages and disadvantages of spitting and swallowing after oral sex. He insists that he squirmed more during those one hundred and fifty minutes than he had ever squirmed before in his entire life and says that what made it worse was the fact that his girlfriend's mother spoke in a rather loud voice. She really did seem to think that this was by far the most interesting subject anyone could talk about around the dinner table.

My reader's girlfriend's father on the other hand apparently took it all quite calmly – maybe he was used to discussions of that type around the dinner table.

Deciding whether to spit or swallow after performing oral sex on a man who has come in your mouth might not sound like an earth shattering decision but to many women it's a real dilemma.

Some worry that the semen they have taken into their mouth may in some way be dangerous and that is, I suppose, the first worry to deal with.

As long as the man is perfectly healthy and is not carrying

Ejaculate may leave the penis at up to 28 mph.

any diseases at all then the semen itself isn't really likely to do any harm once it gets into your mouth. Indeed, there are some who believe that the nutrients in semen can be quite valuable.

It is, however, vital to be careful that the semen doesn't go down the wrong way. It is possible to choke while performing oral sex if you aren't careful and don't concentrate on what you are doing.

Semen isn't going to ruin anyone's diet. At just a few calories a spoonful, semen comes pretty low on the list of fattening products.

So it really comes down to a matter of personal taste.

Some women quite like the taste of semen and feel that swallowing is an important and essential part of oral sex. It is also convenient, of course, because there is no worry about what to do with the semen afterwards.

Other women don't like the idea of swallowing and much prefer to spit the semen out. For them it is important to have a paper tissue handy. If you have to rush out to the bathroom or leap out of bed and find a spittoon – and there aren't many of those around these days in most bedrooms – the atmosphere that has been built up is likely to be destroyed.

If she likes him to come in her mouth then she should try to catch the ejaculate on her tongue since women have choked to death when performing fellatio (very rarely I hasten to add). If she wants him to come in her mouth and wants to swallow but she doesn't like the taste then she could experiment with a deep throat or deep mouth technique, taking his penis to the back of her mouth and allowing him to ejaculate straight down her throat. This is a trick rather akin to sword swallowing and it takes a good deal of practice. Remember the danger of choking and take great care. He should always try to warn her beforehand when he is coming.

If she doesn't want him to come in her mouth then he should

> Men with more than one wife are capable of more erections and more orgasms. Some polygamous men regularly have sex ten times a night.

respect her wish and make sure that he pulls out of her mouth in time. Some women who do not like their partners to ejaculate in their mouths like to watch their partners orgasm and may like to catch the semen in their hands or on their breasts.

Finally, two points.

First, it is important to remember that a number of diseases can be transmitted via oral sex. A condom can provide some protection and unless you know that your partner is free of diseases then you should use one. Diseases can be transmitted from sexual organ to mouth or the other way.

Second, if cunnilingus follows fellatio and kissing in the right order then – in theory at least – result can be conception and, in nine months time, a baby. All that has to happen is that he comes in her mouth, she passes the semen to him in a kiss and he deposits the semen in her vagina from his mouth. Not impossible.

ORGASM (INABILITY TO HAVE)

It is a myth that every woman should orgasm every time she has sex. This myth probably causes more heartache than any other sexual myth. It is supplemented by the modern myth that every woman is entitled to a sequence of orgasms (a multiple orgasm) every time she has sex.

The truth is that the majority of women do not normally have an orgasm during intercourse. Most women only reach orgasm when they masturbate or when their partner supplements vaginal penetration with some form of clitoral stimulation.

The fact that a woman doesn't have an orgasm when she has sex doesn't mean that she is frigid – or that there is anything wrong with her technique or her partner's technique. (And it is worth remembering that most women – and men too – would agree that it isn't necessary to have an orgasm to have good sex. You can enjoy yourself in bed without that final flourish.)

> Sex between consenting but unmarried adult heterosexuals is illegal in nine American states. Oral sex – both giving and receiving – is illegal in 20 American states.

~ Sex ~

Here is my advice for women who have difficulty in reaching orgasm:

1. Tell your partner what you like – and what turns you on. Don't be shy. If some things turn you on – tell him. If other things turn you off – tell him. If you don't tell him – he'll probably never know. At the same time encourage him to tell you what he likes best.
2. Try not to have sex when you are anxious or under pressure. Take the telephone off the hook if you find it difficult to ignore. Try to relax and push your problems to one side before you have sex. If you are preoccupied then your chances of having an orgasm are remote.
3. Do not be afraid to fantasise. Most women find it easier to reach an orgasm if they fantasise. Try reading books with sexy scenes or watching sexy movies if you are not sure what to fantasise about. Don't be worried by your fantasies – however bizarre they may seem. There is a lot of difference between what happens in your fantasies and what happens in real life.
4. Be prepared to let yourself go. Many women find that dressing up for sex (for example, in black stockings and suspenders) turns them on because it turns their partners on. They like feeling exceptionally feminine. You are more likely to reach orgasm if you are enjoying sex. Don't make the mistake of taking ordinary everyday sex too seriously (I am assuming that you are not having sex only to have a baby).
5. If you have difficulty in reaching orgasm during sex try masturbating. If you feel shy about using your hands, or if that doesn't seem to work, try using a vibrator. Then incorporate what you have learned into your love making.
6. Some women may find themselves better able to orgasm if they try this position, based on the missionary position. She lies on her back and he lies down on top of her with his legs in between

---

During Victorian times there were 150,000 prostitutes operating in London (serving a total population of 2,000,000).

her legs. Being a gentleman he takes his weight on his elbows – keeping it off her chest. Next – and this is the movement that really makes all the difference – he slides forwards a little so that he is higher up on her than he was. In this position his pelvis will be over hers and the base of his penis will be rubbing directly against her clitoris. This is why this position works so well. He then takes the weight off his elbows and lowers his chest onto his partner. As he does this his head and shoulders move slightly to one side. It is important that he doesn't let his body slip backwards – remember it is vital for the success of this position that his penis should be pressed against her clitoris – right up against the top of her vagina.

When he starts moving he does so in slow up and down movements – moving his penis a few centimetres at a time and keeping it pressed against her clitoris. He keeps his body firmly pressed against hers – she should keep her legs flat on the bed or floor. She should push up and he should push down.

A slow, rocking motion will probably produce the best results and each stroke should last several seconds. It is the steady rhythmic movement of the penis – with the top of the penis rubbing against the clitoris – which leads to orgasm.

Like everything else in this world this position works best if you practise it as much as you can.

ORGASM (FEMALE)

The first sign that a woman is beginning to respond sexually – and that her body is preparing for intercourse – is when her vagina becomes moist with lubricating fluid. Lubrication usually starts quite quickly – usually within ten to thirty seconds of stimulation. (It is important to note, however, that lubrication of the vagina can result from many other types of stimulus – including: fear, anxiety and general excitement).

> One in twenty men have worn female clothing while having sex with a woman.

The lubrication comes from several sources. Most of it comes from the glands at the entrance to the vagina, but some comes from the walls of the vagina itself. When a woman is aroused, blood enters the tissues around the vagina in the same way that blood flows into the penis of the stimulated man. The fluid that seeps out of the walls of the vagina has come from congested blood vessels.

While this is happening the clitoris is growing – also as a result of blood flowing into the area. The erectile tissue within the clitoris swells in exactly the same way that the erectile tissue in the penis swells. There are, in addition, changes in the breasts in this early phase of sexual excitement. The muscle fibres around the nipples contract with the result that the nipples become erect and the nipples increase in size as blood flows into them. The areas around the nipples – the areolae – become slightly swollen and in some women (particularly women who have never had children) the whole breast is likely to swell.

When a penis enters the vagina the physical presence of the male organ pulls on the labia minora with the result that there is some friction between the part of the labia that covers the clitoris (the clitoral hood) and the clitoris itself. Since the clitoris is packed with sensitive nerve endings – and is already swollen with blood – the response is often fairly fast and quite dramatic. The outer lips – the labia majora – open a little wider and become swollen, moving away from the vaginal entrance in order to give the penis more room. The labia minora also swell a little and the vaginal muscles in the outer part of the vagina expand.

In addition to these very specific changes in and around the vagina there are also some more general changes in a woman's body when sexual intercourse starts. The woman's pulse will increase, her blood pressure will rise and a red flush – rather like a measles rash – will appear on her breasts, chest and upper abdomen. This sort of skin rash can occur in men but it is much com-

---

In a now classic pornographic film made in the USA a famous American film star takes a man's foot inside her vagina.

moner in women – three quarters of whom show some sort of rash during sexual excitement.

Sexual excitement in women (and in men) consists of several phases.

The first phase is one of excitement and arousal.

The second phase is known as the plateau and it is during this phase that the woman's body is prepared for orgasm. The woman's breathing rate increases, her pulse and blood pressure go up even further, any flushing that has already appeared will become more noticeable and more widespread and her muscles will show signs of tension with her face, hands and buttocks showing muscle tension. In the plateau phase of sexual excitement a woman's breasts, nipples and areolae will swell even more than before. Inside the vagina drops of fluid will ooze out from the Bartholin's glands and the tissues in and around the outer part of the vagina will swell. As the vagina tissues swell the vagina will grip the penis more and more tightly. The labia minora will darken in colour – going from pink to purple – and the clitoris will gradually become larger and more elevated.

The woman is now ready for an orgasm – the third and final phase of the excitement process.

There are many myths about just how women have orgasms and where they come from but an orgasm is an orgasm is an orgasm is an orgasm and at the moment of truth it doesn't usually matter terribly where it came from or how it came about. There is, however, much discussion among sex experts about whether an orgasm can be triggered by stimulating the clitoris alone or whether stimulation of the vagina can also trigger an orgasm.

In cold, clinical terms an orgasm is defined as a 'peak of sexual arousal which consists of uncontrollable muscle movements, a tingling, a general feeling of warmth and an indescribable sense of joy and pleasure'. A physiologist once described an orgasm as a

---

> In Europe the average love-making session lasts ten minutes from first caress to final groan.

'mass neuronal discharge, originating in a part of the brain between the amygdala and the hypothalamus'. Technically an orgasm is the same in women as it is in men, and the following seven physical signs may be noticed (but often only by a disinterested observer):

1. A progressive loss of intellectual capabilities.
2. Dilatation of the pupils.
3. An agonised facial expression.
4. Shouting out loud – known as involuntary vocalisation.
5. An increase in the pulse rate (rising to somewhere between 120 and 150).
6. An involuntary heavy thrusting movement of the pelvis.
7. Contractions and tightening of various muscles around the body – resulting in gasping breathing, tightening of the fingers, spreading of the toes and an upward movement of the big toe.

During a woman's orgasm the outer third of her vagina will usually contract rhythmically, too. A mild orgasm may be accompanied by three to five contractions whereas an intense orgasm will probably be accompanied by eight to twelve contractions. The longest recorded series of consecutive contractions is twenty five – lasting for a total of forty three seconds.

When these pelvic contractions take place some women say that they feel as if they are ejaculating. Others simply describe the contractions as a throbbing sensation which makes them feel warm all over.

Despite the fact that the clitoris can be stimulated by the movement of the penis in and out of the vagina, most women do not have their orgasms directly as a result of sexual intercourse but usually need some additional manual stimulation. This inability to orgasm during sex often produces anxiety and guilt among women and men – who often feel that they have failed if they have to resort to such methods.

Three quarters of all men say that their penis hangs on the left hand side.

If a woman is fully aroused and sexually excited before penetration takes place she may be able to reach an orgasm in as little as fifteen seconds. Normally, however, a woman takes rather longer – four and a half minutes from start to finish is average. This is often considerably longer than a man can wait before he ejaculates and so his erection may start to lose its strength long before she reaches her orgasm.

When a woman has an orgasm the muscle tensions that have accumulated will slowly disappear. Blood will slowly flow out of the labia, the clitoris, the nipples and the areolae and all those organs and tissues will shrink back to their normal size. The sexual flush will disappear from the skin (though many women do then begin to perspire – notably on their hands and on the soles of their feet), the vaginal muscles will go back to normal and the clitoris will shrink and fall back downwards again to its previous position. At the same time as all this is happening the opening in the cervix will expand slightly to give the sperm a better chance to swim through into the uterus.

The post ejaculatory depression which affects men so much does sometimes also affect women. It may help a woman who wants to get pregnant because by encouraging her to stay where she is – ideally flat on her back – it ensures that the semen that has been deposited will stay where it is and will not be displaced by any more movement or by muscle contractions resulting from more sexual arousal. Gynaecologists treating women who are trying to get pregnant usually advise them to rest – and to stay flat on their backs – after sex. Standing up merely makes life harder for the sperm.

Women who do not have an orgasm after being sexually aroused may, in addition to being left with a feeling of frustration and a lack of satisfaction, be left with pain and congestion in the pelvic area. The blood vessels which have swollen and filled with

---

> Most people would rather have quite nice sex in a clean house than sensational, mind-blowing, groin-tingling, heart-stopping sex in a dirty house.

blood do not empty quite so quickly when the first stages of orgasm do not lead to the final stage.

ORGASM (MALE)

As soon as a man becomes interested in sex he will usually have an erection. It is the first clear physical sign of arousal and is both difficult to disguise and easy to interpret.

But an erect penis isn't the only sign of sexual arousal: his pulse and blood pressure will rise, his breathing rate will increase, he may acquire a skin flush, his testes will increase in size by as much as fifty per cent and will be pulled higher into his scrotum, his nipples will become erect, the muscles of his face will probably show some signs of tension and his buttock muscles will become tight and tense too.

A few moments before ejaculation a few drops of a clear, sticky fluid will leak out of the end of the penis to moisten the glans and to prepare the way for the flow of semen which should follow. These few drops of fluid may contain some sperm and can, on occasion, lead to a pregnancy.

At about the same time the seminal fluid which contains the sperm will collect in the seminal vesicles which will contract rhythmically, expelling their contents into the urethra at exactly the same moment as the prostate gland contracts and expels its secretions. A bulb in the urethra near the base of the penis more than doubles in size in order to provide the space to store these fluids for a few moments.

Once a male orgasm starts it cannot be stopped.

Strong contractions of the urethra and the prostate gland occur at intervals of just under a second and the semen is forced out through the urethra with a considerable amount of force. Sperm leaves the penis with enough force to travel several feet (the current world record is alleged to stand at 2.6 metres) though it is not al-

---

In 1871 the British Army and Navy spent over £50,000 of official funds on keeping 2,700 prostitutes at naval and military stations around the United Kingdom.

ways possible to measure the force involved in this way. The ancient Hebrews used to believe that if sperm didn't come out forcefully then it wasn't fertile and there is some sense in that.

Sperm that leaves the penis forcefully will be more likely to reach the cervix and therefore the uterus where it will meet an egg. In older men semen leaves the penis with less force and, if unimpeded, is likely to travel a less spectacular distance. Most of the semen is usually forced out in just five or six spurts although the world record is believed to be twenty.

Gradually, the contractions weaken and become less regular. Sometimes a few drops of urine may escape during all this physiological excitement – despite the existence of a valve designed to prevent such an occurrence. This small amount of urine will not do any harm.

Within a few seconds all the available semen will have been forced out of the penis and the ejaculation will be over.

At the moment of ejaculation a man's pulse rate, blood pressure and breathing rate will all reach a peak; any skin flush will deepen; his hands will clench; his facial muscles may go into spasm; his toes will spread and his whole body may become arched. Outwardly, the signs of orgasm in a man are similar to those in a woman.

Soon after the last drop of semen leaves the urethra, the penis, its job as sperm distributor done, will begin to wilt and will lose its size. This process, known as detumescence, usually takes between a few seconds and a few minutes. In some animals small hooks hold the penis in place at this stage so that sexual intercourse will not end abruptly. There is no such aid on the human male organ and sexual interest often subsides rapidly – often giving rise to the complaint that 'he just rolls over and falls asleep as soon as he's finished'.

After ejaculation the blood that has filled the penis and provided it with strength and size leaves.

The average divorced man has 8 sexual partners in the first year after his divorce.

First, the arteries which opened up as the erection developed become constricted again with the result that no more blood can flow into the penis.

And then the blood that is already in the penis – and that has been trapped there – flows out, slowly at first, and then, as the tissues become less and less compressed, more speedily.

The collapse of an erection normally only occurs after ejaculation has taken place, but it can occur if anything unpleasant or frightening happens. A harsh comment, a sudden noise, a pain or a request to paint the ceiling can all lead to an almost instant disappearance of an otherwise satisfactory erection.

As the blood flows out of the penis the testicles begin to shrink and the scrotal sac lowers them down again. Blood flows out of the nipples, which get smaller, and any skin flush slowly disappears. The pulse rate drops, the blood pressure falls and breathing returns to normal. His penis and testicles may be extremely sensitive and tender to the touch.

A man cannot have another erection – or even get very excited sexually – for a while after an orgasm has concluded. This is known as the 'refractory period' and is a stage of the orgasm that women do not have. The length of the 'refractory period' varies according to the individual's age and state of mind. Excitement, guilt or the ordinary stresses of every day life can all have an influence.

In addition to the physical aftermath it is also common for men to feel sad or even depressed after an orgasm, though the likelihood of this happening depends to a large extent upon the nature of the relationship. If the relationship is a satisfying and loving one then the man may be left with a warm, contented, happy feeling. But if the relationship is a one night stand then he may become depressed as he worries about risks and consequences.

It is quite common for men to feel so mentally drained and

One in five men routinely climax in less than two minutes.

so physically exhausted after an orgasm that they have difficulty in staying awake. When young and making love to a new partner for the first time, a man may find it fairly easy to remain alert and interested but when a relationship is a longer established one a man may simply fall asleep.

If an erection does not lead to an orgasm a man will not only be left feeling mentally frustrated but may also feel some pain from prostatic engorgement.

Pain

Only a masochist enjoys sex when it hurts.

There are numerous reasons why sex may be painful: superficial pains and soreness can be caused by vaginal dryness, by allergy reactions, by cuts and sores or by localised infections. Forgotten tampons and other objects accidentally left inside the vagina can cause considerable discomfort. Cystitis is another possible cause of pain. A rigid hymen, an opening made too small after the repair of a tear caused by childbirth and vaginismus can all cause problems. Deeper pains may be caused by fibroids, endometriosis, chronic pelvic congestion (sometimes caused by having sex repeatedly without ever having an orgasm), ovarian cysts, irritable bowel syndrome, a retroverted uterus, a prolapse or an infection of the cervix.

Whenever sex is painful consult your doctor.

Penis

The male sexual equipment is stored outside the body and is, therefore, highly visible to any observer. It consists of a penis and a scrotum, or sack, which holds the two testicles.

Male equipment has two simple jobs to perform: production and distribution.

King Herod slept next to his dead wife Marianne for seven years.

~ Sex ~

The production task involving preparing a large quantity of good quality sperm. Each individual sperm is very small and in order to ensure that there is a fighting chance that an egg will be fertilised it is essential that a huge number of sperm are made. Quality and quantity are the two criteria by which the production department is judged. The production department can sometimes fail to do its job properly but any such failure is usually only identified microscopically. No one is likely to notice if the production department screws up. Production of sperm is carried out in the two testicles which are stored outside the body so that the local temperature doesn't rise too much. The sperm production department won't work properly if the temperature goes too high.

Although no one notices if the production department fails to produce good quantities of well made sperm everyone notices if the distribution department doesn't do its job properly.

The task of the distribution department is to deposit as many of those sperm as possible close to a woman's womb so that they have a decent chance of reaching and fertilising an egg. It is the distribution aspect of the male function that attracts most interest and creates most problems.

The simple problem that the distribution department has to overcome is the fact that the egg waiting to be fertilised is hidden quite deep inside the woman's body. If the sperm were left at the entrance to the vagina they would never get there in time. They would die, exhausted and frustrated, long before they reached their target. Leaving sperm at the entrance to the vagina would be like dumping children twenty miles from the school gates and expecting them to make their own way to school.

To solve the distribution problem the male body uses the penis to put the sperm as close as possible to the target.

In its normal state the male penis is quite limp and flaccid and rather small. It is perfectly adequate for passing urine but as a

---

A recent survey showed that nine out of ten women enjoy being undressed during sex.

tool for entering the female vagina it lacks a single vital quality: rigidity. Try threading a needle with a limp and dangling end of cotton and you'll see what I mean.

There is some available evidence to suggest that many thousands of years ago the male penis may have had a bone in it to make penetration much easier and to solve this distribution problem completely. In France just thirty or so years ago doctors produced X-ray evidence of a male with a small bone inside his penis.

But a bone fixed to the pelvis wouldn't really be practical. God or nature long ago decided to economise with male architecture and so, in addition to serving its vital role as a male sexual organ, the penis also has to function as a discharge tube for urine, and both semen and urine come out through the same opening in the centre of the glans at the end of the penis. A valve ensures that the penis is only used to urinate when it is limp – a man cannot urinate when he has an erection.

But if the penis had a bone in it which way would it point?

If it pointed downwards penetration would be completely impossible in anything other than a few unusual sexual positions. If the penis pointed upwards then every man would be for ever urinating up towards the ceiling.

So, the penis doesn't have a bone in it.

Instead, it behaves quite differently when performing its two very separate functions. When acting as a conduit for urine the penis remains limp. But when being used as a distribution aid for sperm it becomes solid, larger and more erect so that it can be used to deposit sperm safely inside the vagina.

All penises have much the same general structure (whatever their sizes may be). At birth the male penis consists of two clearly defined parts: the shaft and the more sensitive glans. The glans is partly or completely covered by the foreskin, a loose extension of the skin which covers the rest of the penis. Underneath the penis a

---

Middle Eastern males are known to turn female crocodiles on their backs (so that they are helpless) and to then have sex with them.

fairly thin fold of skin – the frenulum – holds the glans to the shaft of the penis. If the frenulum is unusually short it will prevent the penis from becoming properly erect and will lead to premature ejaculation. In well over 90% of male babies the foreskin is tight and difficult to pull down from the glans, but by the time a boy reaches puberty his foreskin will have usually become much looser. When male hormones circulate at puberty the glans pushes out through the foreskin. A number of small glands on the inner surface of the double fold of the foreskin produce a type of lubricating grease which helps to protect the sensitive glans.

For a variety of reasons the foreskin is sometimes removed during an operation known as circumcision but it is important to remember that this apparently useless piece of skin which is so easily removed exists for a purpose. Its job is to protect the glans from irritation and in men who have no foreskin the urethral opening gets gradually smaller and smaller as a result of scarring of the glans. There is, in addition, some evidence that when a man loses his foreskin his glans will become slightly less sensitive.

PENIS SIZE (INCLUDING HOW TO MEASURE A PENIS)

At birth the average erect penis is little more than two and a half centimetres long. By the time a boy reaches the age of twelve his erect penis will probably be about twice that length. It's then that things usually start to improve fairly dramatically. By the age of fifteen the average erect penis is around 12.5 cms (5 inches) long and by full adulthood the average erect penis is between 12.5 and 17.5 cms (5 and 7 inches) long.

One of the very few physical benefits associated with ageing is the fact that the size of an adult penis tends to increase slightly with age – and the length of a fairly ordinary, average sort of penis can increase by as much as 2.5 cm (1 inch) throughout its owner's adult lifetime.

> Chinese men used to believe that eating the warm brains of freshly decapitated criminals would make their penises larger.

The size of the average penis seems to have got slightly bigger over the last century or so. Surveys done in the late nineteenth century showed that the length of the average penis ranged between 7.5 cms and 11.5 (3 and 4.5 inches) cms in length so there seems to have been a healthy increase in the last hundred years or so.

The majority of men are remarkably close to average size and genuine under or over development is relatively rare. There is far more variation in the size of female breasts than there is in the size of male penises.

There may be a considerable change in the size of a penis when it becomes erect and penis size tends to even out rather a lot during the process of erection. A penis that seems particularly small when limp may double or triple its length when erect whereas the increase in length of a penis that is larger when limp may be less noticeable. The length, width and general size of a penis at rest gives absolutely no indication of its potential size when aroused. In some men the main effect of erection is to increase the length of the penis. In others the main effect is to increase the width. In some men an erection has a relatively slight effect on the size of the penis. A penis which is small when limp may, when erect, become larger than a penis which promised much when limp. Nature has her own way of ensuring that her favours are distributed fairly.

Incidentally, it is a myth that you can tell the size of a man's penis by looking at his overall height or the size of his nose or his feet. The height and weight of the owner have little influence on the size of his penis.

To measure a penis you should gently grasp the end of the erect penis between thumb and first finger and lie it along a ruler which has one end pushed gently against the male pubic bone. Measure to the tip of the glans, not to the end of a stretched foreskin. (A quick way to add an inch or more to penis size is to measure the underside down to the scrotum.)

One African tribe used to require young boys to have sex with the dead body of the first antelope they killed.

~ Sex ~

Men worry a great deal about the size of their penises and whatever Freud may say true penis envy is commoner among men than among women. Men worry about the size of their penises about as much as women worry about the size of their breasts (which is very often). Such worries are common among both homosexuals and heterosexuals. A study of one thousand gay men in America showed that over a third thought that the size of a partner's penis was very important. Almost all the homosexuals interviewed – even those who had penises noticeably larger than average – felt that their penises were too small.

Young boys often feel under-endowed when they look around in the school showers. What they do not realise is that boys of a similar age may have reached puberty much earlier and their organs may, therefore, have started to get larger sooner.

Men often feel under-endowed when they look around in the showers after playing squash or football or working out in the gym. What they fail to realise is that each man's view of his own penis is often shortened by an optical illusion when he looks down on it. If two men face one another naked both will almost always think that the other has a considerably larger penis. Some comfort can usually be obtained by looking in a mirror when a more accurate view can be obtained.

Most of these fears are unfounded anyway. There is no correlation between the size of a man's penis and his ability to satisfy a woman sexually. When women do find large penises more exciting it is usually because they look more exciting rather than because they provide more sexual satisfaction. Some women like to admire large penises in the same way that some men like to admire large breasts. The admiration is largely artistic rather than functional.

Occasionally a man may worry that his penis is too big. And some women worry that if a man has too large a penis it may hurt them during sex.

One in three women say they aren't getting enough sex.

Theoretically it is possible that an unusually large penis could hurt a woman but the risk is fairly small since the female vagina can expand and adapt itself to cope with a baby's head (which is rather larger than any penis ever recorded).

The thickness of a penis has far more effect than the length of a penis on a woman's chance of reaching an orgasm during vaginal sex. The unstretched vagina is usually around 10–12.5 cms (4–5 inches) long so the average penis is longer than is necessary to reach the cervix. It is the thickness of the penis which decides how much the labia minora will be moved during intercourse and it is the movement of the labia minora which stimulates the clitoris and produces the female orgasm. Women may find a long, slender penis attractive to look at but a short, fat penis is more likely to provide them with sexual satisfaction.

I constantly receive letters from male readers who are too shy to initiate sexual contact with women they fancy because they fear that they will be rejected or – worse still – laughed at when the partner of their dreams sees how much they've got (or rather how much they haven't got) tucked into their trousers.

The good news is that even if a man does have a slightly smaller than average sized penis he can, by carefully selecting the positions he uses when making love, maximise the amount of satisfaction his partner receives.

See also: Penis (too big) and Penis (too small)

PENIS (TOO BIG)

Theoretically it is possible that an unusually large penis could hurt a woman but the risk is fairly small since the female vagina can expand and adapt itself to cope with a baby's head (which is rather larger than any penis ever recorded).

The only real hazard is that if a penis is exceptionally long it

> Most men admit that they regard at least one of the women they work with to be sexually attractive.

could deposit sperm in the vaginal cul-de-sac behind the cervix. This would make it difficult for sperm to get into the womb and so reduce the chances of the woman getting pregnant.

In addition a very long penis could cause pain by lifting the uterus upwards. On the other hand, if a penis is long enough to touch the cervix during love making it may trigger an orgasm as it does so.

A man with an unusually large organ will need to have a very strong erection. A man with an exceptionally large organ will probably not be able to get away with a half-hearted erection because he will have difficulty in pushing his member between the labia minora into the vagina.

Note that the thickness of a penis has far more effect than the length of a penis on a woman's chance of reaching an orgasm during vaginal sex. The unstretched vagina is usually around 10 to 12.5 cms (4 – 5 inches) long so the average penis is longer than is necessary to reach the cervix. It is the thickness of the penis which decides how much the labia minora will be moved during intercourse and it is the movement of the labia minora which stimulates the clitoris and produces the female orgasm. Women may find a long, slender penis attractive to look at but a short, fat penis is more likely to provide sexual satisfaction.

Women who suddenly find themselves confronted with a sexual partner who has an unusually large penis are often afraid that sex is going to be unpleasant, painful or even dangerous. Male penises do vary a considerable amount in size and a woman who has had a long term relationship with a man with a modest sized organ will often be alarmed when she finds herself face to face with a penis which is larger than she is used to. Incidentally, I think it is probably worth pointing out at this point that just because a penis is unusually large when it is limp that doesn't mean that when it becomes erect it is going to be gigantic. Small penises seem to

---

The term 'gay' was first used to describe homosexuals in Australia in 1920.

enlarge more than larger penises when aroused, with the result that most male organs are roughly the same sort of size when they are erect. It is genuinely unusual for a man to have a penis which is more than a few centimetres longer than normal – although there are a large number of possibly apocryphal stories of men having penises which end up 25 – 30 cms (10 – 12 inches) long. Not surprisingly a woman who has been used to a man with a 12 cm (5 inch) penis is likely to have quite a shock if she finds herself looking at one which is twice the length. I have never heard of a man having a penis which is too long or too thick for sexual intercourse. Don't forget that the vagina can stretch enough to accommodate a baby's head. Problems are really most likely to develop if the man is in too much of a hurry and the woman isn't relaxed or well enough lubricated.

Before having sex with any man a woman should, of course, be properly aroused. And that means plenty of foreplay. The old Australian technique of yelling "Brace yourself Sheila" really isn't enough for most women. If necessary a woman should use some form of artificial lubrication. In the absence of anything more sophisticated the woman's own saliva will do perfectly well.

Any man making love to a woman for the first time will, if he wants there to be a second time, be gentle, cautious and patient and will take care not to hurt his partner. The female partner in a relationship should be entitled to have the last say in how aggressive sex is going to be.

There are of course some women who do have unusually small or tight vaginas – and there are times when the vagina will close up and make it difficult for a penis to enter. (See Vaginismus).

In general the position which is most suitable for women making love to a partner with an unusually large penis is the woman on top position.

She has control over how far the penis goes into her and she

A dancer in a Paris nightclub regularly drinks a full glass of whisky – using only her vagina.

can see what is happening. She can hold his penis as it goes into her and she can lift herself off if sex becomes uncomfortable.

In the basic 'woman on top' position the male partner lies flat on his back and the female partner kneels above him and lowers herself down onto him. This position, the most passive for a man and the most active, aggressive, assertive and dominant for a woman used to be popular in Ancient Greece and has always been very popular in the Orient.

There are a number of variations on the woman on top position. Remember that because this position originated in the East some of the variations are best suited to individuals who are rather smaller and more agile than many Westerners are. Large lovers may find some of these positions painful or impossible or simply unsatisfying.

1. The first and most obvious variation is for her to face away from him. This means that they cannot see one another and cannot kiss. He can't see what is happening and cannot easily touch her breasts. The female partner, however, has even more control than usual. She can still see what is happening and she can touch and fondle his scrotum. She can control the movement on her clitoris by the way she moves.
2. He kneels and then leans back with one or both hands behind him. She faces him and then shuffles her bottom between his thighs so that she can impale herself on his penis. She can drape her legs over his knees. She will have to stretch her arms out behind her to stop herself falling backwards. Neither partner will be able to use their hands and there is relatively little skin contact in this position but both can see exactly what is happening. Since she is still on top she still has control.
3. He lies on his back and she sits astride him as before. The only difference is that she has both legs on the same side and is, therefore, sitting 'side saddle'. She will probably need to balance her-

---

1 in 100 men have had sex with more than 100 different women.

self by putting her arms behind her and taking some of her weight on her hands on the other side of his legs.
4. He kneels and sits up straight. She squats with her thighs parallel to the ground and balances on the balls of her feet. She then lowers herself onto him, holding onto him to keep herself steady. He can put his hands underneath her bottom to help hold her steady. Even though she probably needs to hold onto him she can keep one hand free so that she can fondle him. She still has almost total control.
5. He lies on his side and lifts one leg up into the air. She then kneels astride his lower leg and lowers herself onto him. She is in total control.
6. He lies flat on his back. She gets into the traditional lotus position (with her legs crossed and tucked under her) while sitting on top of him. She can either face him or face away from him. He will be supporting all her weight on one small area of his body but there is a good chance that if she was big enough and heavy enough to hurt him she probably wouldn't have been able to get into the lotus position in the first place.
7. He sits on an ordinary dining chair. Facing him she then sits astride him. Both partners can touch and caress and kiss. This position requires little effort by either partner. She has most control and penetration is not deep.
8. He lies flat on his back on a narrow, long, low table. With one leg either side of the table she lowers herself onto him. Depending on the height of the table she can squat or remain half standing.
9. He sits with his legs apart. She faces him and edges forward and puts her legs around his body. She then sits down onto his erect penis. Both partners can hold and caress and kiss one another.

With a little imagination, ingenuity, agility and patience it is possible to devise many other variations on these simple themes.

One in four women have had sex with more than one partner at a time.

Penis (too small)

Men constantly worry about the size of their penises. It is a common anxiety and one that is, I think, getting commoner. It seems to have become quite fashionable now for some women who want to worry men, or who want to put men down, to talk about how vital it is for a man to have a large penis if he is ever to become a successful lover. In a way I suppose this might be a reaction to the fact that for years women have had to put up with suggestions that men are only interested in women who have large breasts.

There are sexual positions which you can try if you have a female partner who wants the effect of a bigger penis – or if you want to give the impression that your penis is bigger than it is. Do remember however that you should take care with some of these positions because if you use a position which enables you to penetrate a woman too deeply the result may be pain. Even though these positions may not actually make your penis bigger they will make it seem bigger – and to a large extent that is really all that matters.

The whole problem of having a small penis is made infinitely worse by the fact that when a man looks down at his own penis he will almost always think it is unusually small when compared with the male organs he may have seen on other men in the showers at school or the sports club. This is simply a result of the fact that when you look down at something from above it always looks smaller than when you look across at something. If you've been worried because you've been comparing the size of your own penis with the sizes of other penises that you've seen in the showers then I suggest that you go into the bedroom or some other room where you can be alone and where there is a full length mirror, take off all your clothes and try looking at yourself in the mirror. You may well be very pleasantly surprised.

Remember too that if a penis is slightly smaller than aver-

Foreplay between unmarried lovers lasts – on average – 28 minutes. Foreplay between married lovers lasts – on average – exactly half that time.

age the chances are good that when it becomes sexually aroused and becomes erect it will grow rather more than a penis will if it is larger to begin with. In other words the erectile process tends to even out the differences between the sizes of various penises.

If you think your penis is so small that it is genuinely abnormal then you should talk to your own doctor. Don't be shy — doctors get asked about this sort of thing every day.

Men who are dissatisfied with the size of their penises often ask if it possible to have an operation to make their penis larger. I don't recommend any of the procedures I've investigated. I know that some of the claims sound startling but I'm not convinced. And you have to remember that some techniques or operations may involve a certain amount of risk. Men have, for example, asked me if it is possible for them to have silicone injected into their penises to make them bigger. This is certainly something that I would not recommend because I don't know what would happen in the long term. Nor would I recommend having a surgical operation — unless there is a clear failure of development and you are in the very unusual position of having a penis which is genuinely so small that it doesn't function properly. In my view the only really satisfactory way to make a penis bigger is to make it sexually aroused.

If you do have a penis which is smaller than average there are some sexual positions which will make it more likely for you to be able to satisfy a woman who likes a bigger penis. Do remember, however, that you should be careful when using these positions and that you should only try them when you are both eager and willing and prepared to stop if there is any discomfort.

Here are the positions which will help you make the most of a smaller than average penis. I do stress that you should make sure that you do not do anything your partner does not want to try and that you should be prepared to stop or pull back if she wants you to.

Three quarters of women who are divorced or widowed have sexual affairs before getting married again.

~ Sex ~

1. She lies flat on her back while he moves into a kneeling position between her legs. He then put both his hands underneath her buttocks and lifts her up off the bed. She wraps her legs around his waist. He then put his penis into her.
2. She lies flat on her back and lifts her legs straight up into the air so that her feet are pointing at the ceiling. He then kneels and move close to her and she lowers her legs onto his shoulders. He can then put his penis into her. He should be able to achieve deep penetration in this position even if his penis is quite small.
3. She kneels down on the floor – as though she's looking for a contact lens or about to start scrubbing – and he enters her from behind.

It is crucial to remember that the clitoris is the key to female sexual satisfaction. If, when making love, he tries to ensure that his penis rubs against his partner's clitoris, he will dramatically increase the chances of her reaching orgasm.

PHEROMONES

Both men and women produce chemical substances called pheromones which are designed to arouse and stimulate members of the opposite sex and these can be far more stimulating than artificial perfumes. The smells associated with the secretions produced by the vaginas of non ovulating women are far less attractive to men than the smells produced by secretions during ovulation. The production of pheromones is designed to attract men to women at a time when the women are most likely to conceive. If a group of men gather round one woman at a party then it may be that she is ovulating. In order to make the best of your pheromones you should bathe several hours before meeting someone you want to attract in order to remove unpleasant odours and allow the smells of your pheromones to break through.

A woman who married 16 times – to 14 different men – claimed that 5 out of her 14 different husbands broke her nose.

Place (the right)

Most of the time most people make love in the bedroom. But the bedroom isn't always the best place. Sometimes the walls may be too thin. And sometimes a couple may be inhibited by the thought that their every move, every groan and every gasp will be heard by the in-laws or the children. Noisy bed springs and a door that doesn't lock can turn the most affectionate couple into celibates.

If your sex life has been crushed by family life consider getting someone to look after the children for the weekend – and then going away somewhere romantic where you can escape from blocked drains, piles of ironing, demanding children and thin walls.

Alternatively, why not consider an evening of passion in the car? Many couples start their love life in the car but never even consider it after they're married. And yet despite the fact that gear levers and hand brakes are often positioned in such a way that they make excellent contraceptives many couples find making love in the car (in a safe spot) liberating and enjoyable.

Or recapture the magic of your courtship by spending an evening out: a meal in a restaurant and a cuddle in the back row of the cinema.

If you are both bored with your sex life but you have a home of your own then why not consider making love outside the bedroom? Try the kitchen, living room, guest bedroom, hallway, garage or even the garden.

Positions For Sex (finding the best position and the best position for her to reach orgasm)

There are hundreds of different ways for a man and a woman to make love.

In a condition called elephantiasis the human testicles can swell to a size considerably larger than the individual's head.

~ Sex ~

Some positions lend themselves to particular types of movement, some make penetration easier and some make deeper penetration possible. In the 'woman on top' position the woman will find it far easier to rotate her pelvis than in the 'missionary position'. But in the 'missionary position' the man will find that he has a considerable amount of control over how deep his penis enters her.

When a woman sits astride a man she will be able to control the speed and the depth to which his penis enters her and she will have far more say over the way that her clitoris is stimulated. Men may find that in this position the stimulus on the penis is less intense. This means that the 'woman on top' position is particularly useful for men who ejaculate prematurely or for couples who wish to extend the length of their lovemaking.

Most couples have two or three favourite positions and even when they try new positions they may return to their old, well tried positions either because they find that these positions provide most satisfaction or because they have happy memories of their sexual experiences in those positions.

It is worth remembering that:

- Just because you start off having sex in one position it doesn't mean that you have to finish in the same position. Many couples change position several times while making love – first finding a position that she likes, then trying something that he likes.
- There is no such thing as a 'perfect' sexual position. Whatever gives you both satisfaction is right for you.
- Different positions offer different types of pleasure – but not necessarily different degrees of pleasure.
- Past experiences – happy or unhappy – may lead to long lasting preferences for particular sexual positions
- Battles outside the bedroom can lead to battles in the bedroom. If a couple are constantly fighting for dominance in their every-

---

A survey showed that 86% of the graffiti in male toilets is sexual. The same survey showed that only 25% of the graffiti in female toilets is sexual.

day relationship then the fight will probably spill over into the bedroom – with inevitably disastrous results.
- Long-standing attitudes towards sex may make it difficult for some individuals to try particular positions. For example, men who believe that a woman's place is underneath may find it difficult to make love in the 'woman on top' position. And women who have been brought up to believe that a woman should be submissive during sex may find it difficult to take an aggressive role.
- You may be able to discover things about yourself, your partner and your relationship by analysing your favourite sexual position. If she always insists on the 'woman on top' position then she is probably striving to dominate the relationship. If he is only happy with the 'rear entry position' then he is probably aggressive and dominant, and if he is unhappy with the 'woman on top' position then he is probably sensitive about his masculine role.

• The Missionary Position

This position got its name many years ago when a group of white missionaries visited the South Sea Islands in the south west Pacific. The islanders favoured a sexual position in which the man squats while his partner, lying on her back, wriggled her thighs over his and then impaled herself upon his erect penis. When they caught a glimpse of two of the missionaries making love with the woman lying flat on her back and her husband lying on top of her they were highly amused.

Despite the low opinion of the South Sea Islanders, the missionary position is an excellent way to make love and is probably the most widely known and most widely used. Human beings are the only species to have sex looking at one another in the missionary position (most animals use the rear entry position).

The first advantage of the missionary position is that it is

Two men in Lancashire had sex with the same woman for 46 years – making love to her on alternate nights.

easy to get into. You don't have to be a contortionist. You don't even have to be super-fit or super-flexible. She lies down, usually with her legs apart, and he lies down on top of her with his legs inside hers. If a couple are of a roughly similar height then they will be perfectly positioned. He will be able to slide his erect penis into her vagina and they will be able to see one another and to kiss and to hold one another too.

Some women dislike the position if their partner is large or heavy – claiming that even if he takes some of his weight on his elbows they still feel uncomfortable or suffocated.

Some feminists object to the position; claiming that it puts the woman into an inferior and submissive position which is a physical metaphor for society. But such women are very much in a minority. Here are the reasons why women – and men – like the missionary position.

Women like the missionary position because:

1. They like to be controlled.
Some – but certainly not all – of the women who like the missionary position are passive. They prefer to be made love to by a strong man who will make all the moves and who will determine the pattern of movement and the tempo during sex. They like to lie fairly still. The missionary position enables some women to enjoy what is happening to them without feeling that they have too much control over it. Women who tend to feel guilty about sex can enjoy the physical sensations without too many mental anxieties.

2. They find that it gives them a good orgasm.
Many women who like to take a dominant role in sex enjoy the missionary position because it provides their clitoris with the sort of stimulation that enables them to have a satisfying orgasm. A

King Chou-hsin of the Shang dynasty used to like his female partners to wrap their legs around him. He would then carry them about the room balanced on his erection.

woman in the missionary position can set the pace and can respond quite actively. By spreading her legs wide she can move her hips and her pelvis and if she keeps her feet flat on the bed and bends her knees she will be able to thrust herself against her partner. She can use her hands too; reaching behind him to caress or scratch his back and buttocks or reaching down between their bodies to hold his penis or to touch her own clitoris.

3. It enables them to look at their lover.
The missionary position is one of the few positions that enable both partners to look into one another's eyes and to kiss whenever they want to. Many women claim that they get most emotional pleasure out of the missionary position.

Men like the missionary position because:

1. They can be in charge.
Many men feel happiest when they are in control. They like to feel in charge and the missionary position makes them feel masculine, dominant and aggressive. Men who have doubts about their masculinity do not like positions in which a woman takes an aggressive, dominating role and so for them the missionary position is perfect.

2. They can see, touch and caress their partner.
The missionary position enables a man to look at his partner, to fondle her breasts and to kiss her and to look into her eyes.

• The Woman on Top Position

In the basic 'woman on top' position the male partner lies flat on his back and the female partner kneels above him and lowers herself down onto him.

The longest clitoris ever measured was 12 inches long.

~ Sex ~

This position, the most passive for a man and the most active, aggressive, assertive and dominant for a woman used to be popular in Ancient Greece and has always been very popular in the Orient.

Women like the woman on top position because:

1. She can take control.
Being on top enables the woman to control the depth to which his penis enters her and it also gives her a chance to control the speed and rhythm of their love making. She can either move up and down or round and round or from side to side (in France moving from side to side is known as 'travelling on the Lyon mail coach'). She can lean forwards, kiss him, dangle her breasts in front of his face or hold both his wrists above his head so that he is in a submissive position. She can lean backwards and take herself out of reach. She can reach down and touch his penis and she can take herself to orgasm manually; she can stimulate her clitoris and keep herself close to orgasm for long periods of time. Many women claim that they get more – and better – orgasms in this position. Women who like to remain in control, who are afraid of being dominated, who like to be able to move freely, and who want to assert themselves, prefer this position.

2. She can see what is happening.
In this position she can see him enter her. She can choose to allow him to watch.

Men like the woman on top position because:

1. It means less work for them.
Men who have been ill (or who are still ill) prefer this position be-

> A normal healthy male can develop an erection (from limp to hard) in between 3 to 8 seconds.

cause it enables them to hand over the responsibility for active movement to their partner.

2. Being a passive partner is different
Most men are accustomed to taking the lead in sex. They may find taking a passive role to be an exciting and stimulating experiment.

3. They can see exactly what is happening.
The woman on top position is one of the few positions which enable a man to watch a woman as she approaches orgasm. It is one of the positions in which he can touch, kiss, suck and play with her breasts and nipples while making love.

4. Intercourse is usually prolonged.
Men usually find that they need a good erection to enter a woman in this position but once inside intercourse is likely to be prolonged. Men who suffer from premature ejaculation may prefer this position.

• **The Rear Entry Position**

The rear entry position (known to the French as *croupade*) is very popular. It is one of the most natural sexual positions and is the sexual position used by most mammals as the only option. (Only humans experiment with different sexual positions).

She kneels down and supports her shoulders by putting her hands on the floor. Her back should be horizontal to the floor. He approaches her from behind and uses a hand to guide his penis into her. He may be kneeling or squatting or may even sit astride her, like a jockey on a horse. She has no control over what is happening and unless she looks over her shoulder she can see nothing. He can see everything and if he leans forwards he can touch her breasts and her clitoris. It is possible for him to penetrate her very

---

A man in London claimed to have deflowered 70 virgins in a single year.

---

deeply from this position. He can get maximum penetration by sitting astride her and gripping her thighs with his thighs. Deep penetration is so easy in this position that he must be careful not to push too hard or he may hit an ovary – which can be extremely painful.

If she finds this position tiring or uncomfortable she can build up a pile of cushions or pillows beneath her. Or she can kneel on the floor and rest her arms on a bed or chair. The lower her head the deeper he will be able to penetrate her.

Women like the rear entry position because:

1. She has no control
For women this is the most submissive and impersonal of positions. She cannot see her partner and she has no control over what happens. Women who like to maintain an emotional distance or who like to feel 'used' during sex prefer this position to any other – as do women who enjoy deep penetration.

Men like the rear entry position because:

1. They have control
For men this is probably the most aggressive of all positions. It is a position which is widely used by Eskimos where the lack of face to face contact is considered an advantage because men traditionally loan out their wives to honoured guests. Men who prefer to initiate sex and who like to dominate prefer this position to any other.

• The Side by Side Position

Making love side by side is the most democratic of positions. Both partners face one another and because both pairs of legs have to

> Only 40% of men who regularly go to church enjoy sex.

be entwined to make penetration possible there is an inevitably strong skin contact. Neither partner is dominant and neither is submissive. Both partners can touch and caress and kiss one another. This position is peaceful, restful and physically undemanding.

Factors which influence the choice of position

1. Physical problems
If she suffers from backache, or he has bad arthritis in his knees, then there will be a natural, physical restriction on the available positions. There is no point at all in even trying a sexual position which is painful for one or both partners.

2. Weight
If one partner is much heavier than the other then both partners will probably be happier with a position in which the lighter partner is on top. For example, if the man is much heavier than the woman then the missionary position will be less suitable than the woman on top position.

3. Pregnancy
Positions which put least strain on the woman's abdomen are advisable. Rear entry positions, side by side positions and woman on top positions are all much better than the missionary position for pregnant women.

4. Size of sexual organs
Positions in which deep penetration is inevitable will probably not be suitable if he has an unusually large penis and she has an unusually small vagina. On the other hand if she has an exceptionally spacious vagina and he has a particularly small penis then a deep penetration position will probably be useful.

Three out of four men describe themselves as 'very good' lovers.

---

5. Fears and hang ups
There is no point in choosing a position that appeals to one of you if the other half of the partnership is terrified or embarrassed. The golden rule of happy sex is that you should never do – or even try – anything that both of you are not entirely happy about.

6. Her ability to reach an orgasm
If a woman has a great deal of difficulty in reaching an orgasm during normal intercourse then it is sensible either to choose a position in which the clitoris receives the greatest amount of natural stimulation or to choose a position in which it will be possible for one or both partners to touch the clitoris during intercourse.

7. His ability to maintain a firm erection
Some positions need a really firm erection – others can be managed successfully with an erection that is only moderately firm.

8. Her need to dominate
Some women are only really satisfied by a sexual position in which they can take an aggressive, dominating role. Such women usually prefer woman on top positions – and usually prefer to remain active during sex, rather than passive.

9. His need to dominate
Some men feel uncomfortable if they are not in a dominating and aggressive position during sex.

10. Her need to be dominated
Some women only feel comfortable during sex if they know that their partner is in charge.

Most men believe that job satisfaction and a good car are more important than a hot sex life.

11. His need to be dominated
Less commonly, some men feel more comfortable when the woman they are making love with takes charge.

12. A desire to find a position in which both partners can see what is happening
Some people are turned on by being able to see what is going on – in other words to see their sexual organs in action.

13. A desire to be able to kiss
Some people feel the need to kiss during sex. Without kissing they feel that sex becomes too impersonal and too clinical.

14. A desire to see one another's bodies
In some positions the two partners face in opposite directions. Visual contact disappears completely. Some men and women strongly dislike this type of sex and prefer to be able to see one another.

15. A desire for maximum skin contact
Many people like to be in touch with their partner's bodies during sex. Skin contact makes sex more intimate and more enjoyable.

16. A desire to share everything
Some couples prefer positions in which all aspects of the physical relationship can be shared.

17. His desire to touch her breasts
Men are often aroused by being able to touch their partner's breasts.

18. Her need to touch her clitoris
Because many women can only orgasm if they masturbate, positions in which the woman can touch her own clitoris are often popular.

A couple in Rotherham claim to have made love in over 100 different telephone boxes.

~ Sex ~

19. A need for contact that is exclusively genital
There are some positions in which contact is (almost) exclusively genital.

20. A desire for prolonged intercourse
If he suffers from premature ejaculation – or both partners want their love making to last – then they may want a position in which their orgasms are likely to be delayed.

Pregnancy (fear of)

Neither partner will be able to relax or to enjoy a proper sexual relationship if either one is worried about an unwanted pregnancy.

See also: Contraception

Premature Ejaculation

Some experts say that any ejaculation which happens before both partners are ready for it is premature. Others argue that a man is a premature ejaculator if he cannot withhold ejaculation long enough for his partner to have an orgasm fifty per cent of the time. A third group of experts say that a man is a premature ejaculator only if he cannot stop himself ejaculating for at least a minute after entering his partner. (One in eight men normally require no more than six movements of their penis before they ejaculate – and cannot delay ejaculation for more than six movements). A fourth group say that a man is only a premature ejaculator if he ejaculates before he can get his penis into his partner's vagina. And a fifth group say that a man is a premature ejaculator if he ejaculates before he can get his penis into his partner's vagina or he ejaculates the moment he enters her.

In the 19th century a prostitute called Laura Bell gave her husband a £250,000 dowry – her earnings from just one of her clients.

Premature ejaculation occurs mainly in younger men and tends to disappear after the age of thirty when the reflexes become duller. It is so common that at least one half of all men ejaculate too quickly the first time they make love to an attractive new partner (though the second attempt is usually much more successful).

Premature ejaculation is primarily a psychological problem rather than a physical one. It is commonly caused by over-enthusiasm, great expectations, excitement and anxiety. Over-eagerness to please is probably the commonest cause, and anxiety about it happening is almost certain to make it worse.

Facts about premature ejaculation

1. When man lived in the wild, premature ejaculation was something of an asset. In the days when men were eaten alive by wild animals a man who took a long time over sex might find himself being eaten before he could procreate. A man who took too long to ejaculate probably didn't father too many children.
2. It is more common among men who do not have sex very often.
3. It seems to be common among men who masturbate a great deal.
4. It is also sometimes said that whereas a meat diet tends to increase a man's chances of becoming a premature ejaculator a vegetarian diet makes it unlikely.
5. Some observers claim that premature ejaculation is more common among male horse riders and motor cyclists though, as far as I know, no one has come up with any valid explanation for this observation.
6. Men sometimes ejaculate prematurely if they feel that their partner regards sex as an unwelcome imposition.
7. Sometimes men whose partners have just given birth will ejacu-

---

A man produces 72 million sperm a day – enough to populate the entire world in three months.

late prematurely. Psychologists argue that they feel bad about having sex with a woman who is a mother and so (driven by a subconscious force) try to get it over with as quickly as possible.

8. Men who were starved of affection and love when young are often premature ejaculators.
9. Some women fear that if their partner ejaculates prematurely it must be because he doesn't 'fancy' them – or because he is thinking about some other woman. Both theories are wrong.
10. Many men who worry that they are ejaculating prematurely last between one and six minutes after penetration. This is within normal limits. It is rare for a man to be able to last for the ten minutes or so that the average woman needs to reach an orgasm. Most women who do reach orgasm directly and solely through intercourse need at least ten minutes of solid, hard thrusting. That sort of requirement can make sex far too much like hard work for many men. It is probably better for both partners to accept that she is unlikely to reach orgasm through sex alone and better if he helps her reach orgasm through manual or oral clitoral stimulation or if she helps herself to an orgasm through masturbation. (This problem is not unique to human beings. Male chimpanzees routinely reach orgasm in about thirty seconds and their partners usually get sexual satisfaction by having sex with as many males as possible – or necessary – one after the other).

Nine Tips for Men who want to conquer premature ejaculation

1. Try wearing a condom during intercourse. The condom will reduce the stimulation which hastens an orgasm.
2. Try using an anaesthetic cream – available from any good pharmacy. This should have the same effect as wearing a condom.

One in 100 women have had sex with 20 or more men.

3. Most men find that their second erection disappears much less speedily than their first. So, if the first ends quickly in a premature ejaculation and disappointment for both partners wait a while and then try again.
4. It is sometimes possible to extend the life-span of an erection by distracting yourself with some sexually unstimulating thought. Some men try to do mathematical problems or try to work out difficulties at work while making love in order to prolong the life of an erection.
5. Tense your buttock muscles while making love – this should help to delay the moment of orgasm.
6. Satisfy your partner orally or manually before you enter her. Knowing that she will not be left frustrated – however quickly you ejaculate – should help reduce the pressure and enable you to last far longer.
7. Gently pull down your testicles before penetration and during intercourse. Prior to ejaculation the testicles normally rise slowly towards the base of the penis. By pulling them (very gently) in the opposite direction you may be able to delay orgasm.
8. Many young men learn to come quickly – possibly because they are frightened of being discovered while masturbating. You may be able to learn to come more slowly by trying to delay your orgasm as long as possible while masturbating.
9. Recruit your partner's help. She should sit on the bed with her back resting against the bed-head. You lie near to her so that she can hold your penis in her hand. She then masturbates you. The moment you feel that you are about to ejaculate you should tell her. She should then gently squeeze your penis at the point where the glans meets the shaft, holding it still for around five seconds. This should stop the ejaculation. You should then both relax for a minute or so before she resumes masturbating you. Using this technique should enable you

---

Four out of ten married women have tried anal sex.

gradually to build up your resistance – and your confidence in your resistance. Once you are satisfied that you are making good progress with this technique begin practising inside your partner's vagina. She should take the 'woman on top' position and you should keep quite still. She then moves, slowly and carefully, and you tell her if you feel that you are close to coming. She should then keep still for a few moments until you feel that it is safe for her to continue. After practising this technique for a while most men notice a considerable improvement.

REPULSION

It may sound cruel to mention this but it's a fact of life and to ignore it would be pointless.

As we get older and more secure and settled in a relationship we tend to take things for granted. We often let ourselves go.

When we are young we make a real effort to look at our best. We buy fashionable clothes and we dress carefully. We look after our hair and our skin and we try to control our weight.

But as the years go by these things become less and less important.

He may become fat, bald and scruffy. With his shoulders covered in flakes of dandruff. He may not bother to shave at the weekends.

She may become comfortably 'plump'; dressing always in sensible clothes and making no effort with her hair or her make up unless she is going out to meet friends.

You may not think that these things matter. And in some relationships they do not. True love is often blind.

But if a relationship is rocky or under pressure appearances can be extremely important.

The average American prostitute has sex with 694 men in an average year.

Retarded Ejaculation

Retarded ejaculation is the opposite to premature ejaculation – and it is far less common.

Men may have difficulty in reaching orgasm for several reasons:

1. They have deliberately tried to hold back (either in the hope that their partner will reach her orgasm or in an attempt to avoid the risk of making their partner pregnant). Afterwards, when they try to ejaculate they find that they can longer come and that they have 'gone past the point of no return'.
2. They feel guilty about ejaculating. If a man is worried for any reason (he may be making love to a woman who is not his wife or he may be worried about making his partner pregnant) then he may have difficulty in obtaining an erection or, if he has an erection successfully, he may have difficulty in ejaculating.
3. They may have drunk too much alcohol or taken too many reflex dulling pills.

Men who suffer from retarded ejaculation can sometimes help themselves by fantasising, by persuading their partner to try a different position, or by masturbating to a position close to orgasm and then continuing with normal sexual intercourse.

Sometimes the female partner may be able to help by using a different technique, by providing manual stimulation or by initiating fellatio. Retarded ejaculation is a problem which most commonly affects men over the age of fifty.

Rhythm Method

If fertilisation is to take place the sperm and the egg must be in roughly the same place at roughly the same time. Since the egg is released at ovulation, which normally takes place roughly midway

---

Sexy star Mae West did not start her film career until she was 40 years old.

between menstrual bleeds, it is possible to estimate when conception is most likely to take place. And by the same reckoning it is possible to estimate when conception is least likely to take place.

An egg can live for about two days and sperm have a practical life-span of a similar length. Theoretically, that means that if sperm can be kept out of the vagina for two days each side of ovulation then there is unlikely to be a pregnancy.

Ovulation normally happens between twelve and sixteen days before the beginning of a menstrual bleed. So those who favour the rhythm method suggest that sex be avoided between the tenth and the twentieth days of the cycle – as long as the cycle is regular.

Some experts claim that you can tell when ovulation takes place by measuring body temperature. The body temperature of a woman goes down slightly and then up slightly when an egg is released so daily temperature readings will, in theory at least, help identify the point of ovulation. Another technique depends on the fact that the mucus in the vagina becomes wetter and more transparent at ovulation.

I think the rhythm method is too risky to be relied upon.

Scrotum and Testicles

The scrotum, which contains the two testicles, hangs below and behind the flaccid penis. The two testicles normally hang at different heights, with the left one lower than the right. There is no complex physiological reason for this: it is simply to stop them knocking into one another. The scrotum is a wrinkled sac of skin which is flexible and extremely sensitive to touch, sexual stimulation and temperature changes.

The purpose of the scrotum is to enable the testicles to hang outside the body since they are extremely vulnerable to heat. When the outside temperature rises too much the skin of the scrotal sac becomes looser – enabling the testes to move further away from

> Cleopatra is said to have performed oral sex on a hundred Roman noblemen in a single night.

the body and therefore remain cooler. When the outside temperature drops the scrotum contracts, pulling the testes closer to the body so that they can get warm. You can see this scrotal activity when a man gets into a warm or a cold shower.

In a male baby the testicles develop inside the body and usually move down into the scrotum before birth but occasionally one or both testicles will fail to descend properly. This problem, which affects roughly one in every twenty boys, is called cryptorchidism and either hormone treatment or surgery may be needed to ensure that the testicles do eventually descend into their rightful positions. If the testicles stay inside the body for too long the high temperature can kill the sperm producing tissues and eventually produce infertility.

Fear and sexual excitement can have the same effect on the testicles as cold weather. In children the testicles may go right up inside the body during moments of terror. Some Japanese fighters can still do this and the trick is useful for professional fighters and wrestlers.

The two smallish, egg shaped testicles inside the scrotum have two clear tasks: to produce sperm and to produce male sex hormones. Each testicle is attached to an epididymis where sperm are stored as they mature and two tubes, the vas deferens, which carry the sperm from the testes to the penis. En route, on each side of these tubes, there are storage sacs called seminal vesicles where mature sperm can be stored. Alongside the vas deferens are the glands which produces the fluid which nourishes the sperm during and after ejaculation.

Semen

Semen is whitish, with a yellowish tinge, and an average ejaculate contains around 5mls (about a teaspoonful). The record amount produced during a single ejaculate is alleged to be two soup-spoon-

---

Porpoises enjoy group sex.

fuls (though there has been relatively little research into this). Men who want to obtain a more copious ejaculate can do so by masturbating nearly but not quite to orgasm an hour or so before sex. This increases the amount of prostatic secretion – and therefore the quantity of semen.

The primary constituent of semen – the fluid produced when a man ejaculates – is sperm. Men produce sperm all the time and the seminal vesicles or storage sacs inside their testicles are full of it. On an average sort of day a healthy man will produce around 90 million sperm – enough to populate North America in half a week or the whole of northern Europe in a whole week. Sperm production is fast and after having sex a normal, healthy man's sperm storage sacs will be full again in just two or three days. If a man doesn't have sex regularly then his sperm producing skills will diminish as will his body's production of testosterone (the male hormone) and therefore his sexual drive.

But although sperm are the most important constituent of semen they aren't the only constituent, and semen contains many different ingredients which together give it its well known horse-chestnut pollen smell and salty taste. There are proteins, sugar, vitamin C and secretions from the prostate gland which stimulate the production of sperm. Semen is so rich in nutrients that in some African tribes it is collected during initiation ceremonies and afterwards used as a remedy for a wide variety of ailments. In many primitive societies women regard semen as a precious food stuff and today numerous scientists claim that semen contains ingredients which can improve a woman's physical and mental health. It seems that some of the ingredients of semen can be absorbed into her body after sex and may help improve her breathing and help control her blood pressure. Two substances contained in semen – histamine and serotonin – are believed to have a useful effect on the womb and its muscles.

> Most men and women believe that true love comes only once in a lifetime.

When semen leaves a young man's penis it will be travelling at just under 30 miles per hour but with age the force of the ejaculation falls.

Sexually Transmitted Diseases

Anyone who has sex is, theoretically at least, exposed to the risk of contracting a sexually transmitted disease. There are about twenty five different sexually transmitted diseases (though if you wanted to count all the diseases that could be transmitted during intercourse you would have to include diseases such as tuberculosis, influenza, chicken pox and measles).

The majority of sexually transmitted diseases are caused by bacteria, parasites, yeasts, viruses, chlamydiae, fungi and mites. The symptoms of infection include rashes, swellings, urinary difficulties (such as bleeding, frequency and pain), soreness, itching, discharges that have increased, changed or become smelly, lumps, ulcers and warts. It is possible for some sufferers (particularly women) to catch a sexually transmitted disease without developing any symptoms.

The commonest symptoms are sores, ulcers and a discharge although the picture is made more confusing by the fact that sexually transmitted diseases are often passed on in groups and when one individual catches several sexually transmitted diseases at the same time the symptoms are, inevitably, confusing.

The sexually transmitted diseases that are most commonly passed on are probably candida, trichomonas, non specific urethritis, gonorrhoea and warts, although herpes and AIDS undoubtedly attract most publicity.

The only ways to avoid the risk of contracting a sexually transmitted disease are either to avoid sex completely, to make sure that you only ever have sex with virgins or to remain totally faithful to someone who is free of disease and who remains totally faithful to you.

During the 18th century a popular whore called Kitty used to charge £20,000 a night for sex.

~ Sex ~

A less certain way to protect yourself and to minimise your risk of contracting an unwanted disease is to make sure that you always use some form of mechanical contraception (preferably a condom), to pass urine immediately after sex (that helps by washing away some potential infections) and (also immediately after sex) to wash yourself with soap and water.

If you have any symptoms of a sexually transmitted disease you should seek medical advice straight away. If you do not have symptoms but suspect that you could have contracted an infection you should go for a check-up. Most sexually transmitted diseases can be dealt with far more effectively when treated early.

Note: Do take care when using public lavatories. It is possible to pick up some sexually transmitted diseases from infected toilet seats.

See also: Chlamydia, Herpes, Gonorrhoea, Syphilis, Thrush, Trichomonas

Slavery

It costs £35 to buy a female slave in northern Sudan. In South East Asia prices are much higher: nearly 250,000 women and children are sold each year at prices up to £6,250 each. Altogether around one million women and children are bought and sold annually in the sex trade. Western governments allow this to happen because the slave trade does not seem to have an adverse effect on the supply of oil.

Spermicidal Creams

Chemicals which kill sperm can be bought as creams, pessaries, tablets, foams and aerosols. They are messy and of doubtful effectiveness although some doctors recommend their use with condoms. By themselves spermicidal substances are probably too much of a

---

A 26 year old man in Coventry claims to have had sex with 100 different women – all called Jane.

gamble to be regarded as an effective or reliable means of contraception.

STERILISATION

Of a man:
Known as a vasectomy this operation is also very simple. Using a local anaesthetic the surgeon closes the tube down which sperm travel from the testes to the penis. Afterwards, although there are no sperm in the semen there is no visible difference and no other effects. It usually takes ten or twenty ejaculations to get rid of waiting sperm and men are usually advised to have two tests done to make sure that their semen is free of sperm. Reversing the operation is difficult.

Some experts are now investigating the possibility that performing a vasectomy may affect the long term health of the individual concerned.

Of a woman:
The gynaecologist makes a small cut in the woman's abdomen and then cuts or removes parts of both tubes and seals them. The procedure is quick and involves a very short hospital stay. The operation is usually effective but difficult to reverse. Because it does not involve the removal of any hormone producing organs it does not affect the woman's feelings, body or sexual drive at all. Since an egg may be waiting in the womb a woman should take her usual precautions until she has a period.

SYPHILIS

Although syphilis used to be the most feared of all sexually transmitted diseases it is today relatively rare.

It usually begins with a painless sore that looks rather like an

---

> One in five women don't like sex because it is messy.

ulcer and which usually appears on the penis or the outside of the vagina. The patient will probably also have a flu like illness – together with swollen glands. The first symptoms of syphilis usually appear anything from nine to ninety days after having sex with an infected partner.

If caught early, syphilis can be treated effectively with antibiotics.

The real danger is that if syphilis goes untreated it can produce heart or brain disease twenty or thirty years later. It is this which makes syphilis one of the most horrifying of all the sexually transmitted diseases.

Thrush

Its proper name is candidiasis though its also known as moniliasis and its millions of sufferers know it as thrush.

And it's on the increase.

Tens of thousands of women get if for the first time every week.

Hundreds of thousands – possibly millions – are long term sufferers.

Although it isn't necessarily transmitted by sex (the fungus that causes it can just start to grow) it often is and it's one of the commonest sexually transmitted diseases around.

If you haven't yet discovered the agonies of having thrush the chances are that you will.

The bug that causes the infection isn't particularly rare. Most people have the candida albicans fungus living on their skin or somewhere else in their bodies.

But it's when the fungus starts to grow out of control that it causes problems.

Theoretically, the candida fungus can grow almost anywhere, but like most fungi the infection that causes thrush prefers some-

---

An American got married 20 times – though he married two of the women twice each so he only had 18 different wives.

where soft, moist, warm and dark. And that means that the vagina is the place most likely to be targeted.

The first symptom of thrush is usually a white, itchy discharge. Sex becomes painful, uncomfortable and unpleasant and the itching can be unbearable. Thick, white patches often appear around the outside of the vagina.

The chances of a candida fungal infection developing are increased when the naturally rather warm and moist area of the vagina is made unnaturally warmer or moister. Wearing nylon underwear, tights or close fitting trousers all make it easier for the candida fungus to grow.

But it isn't only what you wear that determines your susceptibility to thrush:

- The change in circulating oestrogens that occurs during pregnancy or when a woman takes the contraceptive pill can also encourage thrush to develop.
- Eating too much sugar makes the environment even better.
- Being overweight means that fatty folds around the outside of the vagina keep the area unusually moist and warm.
- Taking antibiotics upsets the natural balance of bugs and makes thrush more likely.
- Scratches and skin abrasions can also increase the likelihood of thrush developing.
- Inserting a tampon with dirty hands can also put up your chances of developing the infection.

There are many things you can do to reduce your chances of contracting thrush – or to increase your chances of getting rid of it.

Good local hygiene is important, but it isn't necessary to use antiseptics or deodorants; indeed, such products can increase your problems by irritating the area. Skirts, stockings and no underwear are much better for keeping the area well 'aired'.

A woman's nipples become up to half an inch longer and a quarter of an inch wider when she is sexually aroused.

~ Sex ~

Once a candida infection develops there are several things you can do.

To start with do visit your doctor – he may prescribe an antifungal cream or pessaries. He may also want your partner to have a course of treatment since infection can be passed between the two of you during sex.

Some women have reported a reduction in symptoms after dipping tampons in plain yoghurt and inserting them into the vagina. Yoghurt contains the lactobacilli bacteria which compete with and often oust the infection.

TIME (THE RIGHT TIME FOR SEX)

Television and electricity have ruined sex for most people. Non stop TV encourages us to stay up late and electricity enables us to keep warm without having a cuddle. It's hardly surprising that the biggest jump in the birth-rate occurs nine months after every major power cut – when people discover the joys of things they'd forgotten.

Couples who try to make love late at night after a long evening in front of the TV set and an even longer day at work often discover problems. He'll probably have difficulty in getting a good erection and if he does then he'll either ejaculate quickly or not at all. And he'll be so tired that he'll fall asleep whether she's satisfied or not.

When a couple make love last thing at night after a long and tiring day the chances are high that they will both end up disappointed and frustrated.

The early morning is often a much better time.

Sexual desire is often higher in the mornings and both partners may find it easier to get aroused. Best of all is a morning at the weekend when there's no rush to get to work.

If you're worried about the children wandering in solve that

The oldest recorded sex offender was 90 years old when he was arrested.

---

problem by putting a lock or bolt on the bedroom door.

If early morning just doesn't seem right try going to bed earlier on in the evening. If you can't bear the thought of missing the TV and you don't have a video recorder plan your love making around the programmes you want to watch. Get a friend to look after your children for an hour or two – and return the favour another night.

Trichomonas

Since it produces a nasty vaginal discharge trichomonas is sometimes confused with thrush. The difference is that the discharge associated with trichomonas is usually yellowish green and invariably smells. There is usually some redness and soreness around the vagina too. Trichomonas, like thrush, makes sexual intercourse extremely sore and uncomfortable. Although trichomonas is commonly transmitted through sex it can be picked up from infected towels and lavatory seats. If you think you could have this – or any other vaginal infection see your doctor for the appropriate treatment.

Urethra

Just below the clitoris, at the top of the vestibule, is the opening of the urethra – the tube which allows the bladder to get rid of urine. Strong sphincter muscles which can close together very tightly ensure that urine only flows out of the bladder and down the urethra when it is appropriate but sometimes these muscles may relax a little during sexual arousal with the result that a few drops of urine may leak out. This may be embarrassing but it not harmful. Women who notice this problem can usually avoid it by emptying their bladders before having sex.

One in three boys aged 16 or less claim to have been fellated by a girl. A similar percentage claim to have returned the favour.

Vagina

The vagina has three functions: to let the penis in (so that sperm can be deposited as close to the womb as possible), to allow a baby out and to provide an escape route for the monthly menstrual flow.

The vagina lies directly underneath the urethra and is a rather larger opening (though it is not unknown for the sexually inexperienced to mistake the urethral opening for the vagina with disastrous consequences which include infertility and incontinence). The vaginal opening leads into a muscular tube which stretches backwards and upwards towards the uterus or womb. In young girls who are still virgins the opening of the vagina is often partly (and sometimes completely) sealed by the hymen – a thin sheet of skin which usually dissolves and disappears as a girl grows, leaving remnants around the vaginal entrance.

In some societies the existence of a hymen is regarded as evidence that a girl is still a virgin and a bridegroom expects his new bride to suffer some pain as he stretches and then splits her hymen. A few spots of blood on the bridal sheet are expected and the sheet is then held up to the guests at the wedding reception so that they can see both that the bride was a virgin and that the marriage has been consummated.

These days, however, most brides, whether or not they are sexual virgins, have little or no hymen left by their wedding night. The membrane may be split during bicycle or horse riding, during gymnastics or aerobics or by the use of tampons during menstruation. It is not unknown for cosmetic surgeons to be asked to repair and reinstall a tattered hymen. On rare occasions the hymen may be extremely thick and may need to be surgically pierced if consummation of the marriage or the relationship is impossible.

Just inside the vagina there are two small glands (one on each side) known as Bartholin's glands which have the job of secreting fluid during sexual excitement in order to moisten the vagi-

---

A porn star in the USA specialises in having vaginal sex with two men at the same time.

nal entrance. This fluid is needed to make it easier for the penis to enter the vagina. Occasionally the Bartholin's glands may become infected and swollen.

In addition to the secretions from these glands the walls of the vagina also produce lactic acid which helps to kill off any bugs which might get in from the outside world. Because the inside of the vagina is warm and moist and dark it is an excellent breeding ground for infections of all kinds. The production of lactic acid increases during a woman's reproductive years so that any risk of infection is kept to a minimum during the time that pregnancy might follow intercourse. Before puberty and after the menopause the production of lactic acid secretions falls and in addition to an increased risk of infection there is also more likely to be soreness, dryness and pain during intercourse.

The amount of moisture inside the vagina is increased by sexual excitement but it is not just sexual excitement which has this effect. Happiness, fear and nervousness can all increase the quantity of secretions being produced in the vagina. There is also a slight increase in the amount of vaginal secretion before a menstrual period and a reduction during menstruation and this means that sex during a period may be dry and rather painful. During sexual intercourse the vagina produces more secretions.

The first third of the vagina is made up of a strong ring of muscles which enable the vagina to remain closed when it is not in use and which give its owner the ability to grasp anything that happens to be inside it quite tightly. When these muscles are exercised they can be remarkably strong. Night club entertainers sometimes develop their vaginal musculature to such an extent that they can perform quite remarkable tricks – firing table tennis balls off in all directions or appearing to smoke a cigarette by drawing the smoke into the vagina. More usefully and more commonly these muscles can be developed to improve a woman's sexual skills.

French writer Georges Simenon, the creator of Maigret, claimed to have had sex with 10,000 women.

~ Sex ~

The overall size of the vagina is a subject of some concern both to men and to women. In some tribes in Africa a man who is looking for a new wife will examine her first to check out the size and depth of her vagina. He may also want to see how well padded her mount of Venus is and to check on the size of her labia. Some women worry that their vaginas will be too small to accommodate an erect penis. This fear is usually groundless since the vagina can stretch large enough to accommodate a baby's head. Other women, who may have given birth to several children, worry that their vaginas may have become too spacious. This fear is also groundless since the muscles within the vaginal walls can be strengthened to enable a woman to hold onto a penis of quite modest proportions. The only real risk is that if a woman has a very small vagina and her partner has a very large penis then he may penetrate so far that the tip of his penis knocks into an ovary during sex. Since ovaries, like testicles, are well endowed with nerve endings this can be very painful.

The muscular walls inside the vagina are covered with a membrane. There are remarkably few nerve endings.

VAGINA (DRY)

One in five pre-menopausal women (and considerably more menopausal women) complain that their vaginas are dry – and make sex uncomfortable.

There are several possible causes.

Fear is one possibility (the production of lubricating substances goes down when a woman is afraid) but a lack of proper preparation is even more likely. A longer period of foreplay will usually solve the problem.

If the amount of natural lubrication remains too low oils and jellies can be bought from the pharmacy. Saliva is the cheapest and most readily available lubricant.

Attila the Hun died while having sex
with a blonde.

Vagina (lax)

When a woman has a baby her pelvic and vaginal muscles are put under a considerable strain – inevitably, they have to stretch to let the baby through. It is hardly surprising that those muscles often lose some of their tone and strength.

When this happens a woman may complain that she no longer gets as much satisfaction from sex as she got before. Her partner may complain that he finds sex less satisfying too. The main problem will be that the vaginal muscles will be less able to grip the penis tightly when it enters. As a result there will be less stimulation for him and less likelihood that her labia minora will pull down on her clitoris to take her to (or at least towards) orgasm.

By deliberating exercising the muscles in and around the vagina it is possible to regain vaginal muscle tone.

Here's how:

1. The muscles that control your vaginal walls also control the flow of urine from your bladder. Begin your exercises by sitting on the lavatory with your legs apart and your arms resting on your thighs. Force a little urine out of your bladder. Stop almost immediately, as soon as the stream of urine has started. Use the muscles around your vagina to stop the urine flow. For the next few minutes continue to pass teaspoonfuls of urine in short bursts, contracting your muscles to regulate or control the flow.
2. After practising like this you should be able to contract and relax the relevant muscles without needing a flow of urine to show you that you are succeeding.
3. Try exercising the same muscles while you are lying flat on your back on your bed. Undress first and make sure that the bedroom is warm and that you will not be disturbed. Put a pillow under your bottom.
4. Moisten one clean finger and place it gently inside your vagina.

> Native Australians regularly have sex five times a night – sleeping between each performance.

If you have any difficulty in doing this, lift up your knees and put your feet flat on the bed. While the finger is inside you, try squeezing hard with the muscles around your vagina. You should be able to feel the muscles contracting. Then let the muscles relax and go loose. If you repeat this exercise frequently you should be able to strengthen your vaginal muscles.
5. Without having a finger in your vagina try bearing down – as though you were trying to push a baby out of your vagina. Then, try moving the muscles the other way – so that if there was anything in the front of your vagina it would be sucked inwards.
6. Once you have tried this exercise a few times you'll know what it feels like and you will be able to exercise whatever you are doing and wherever you are. You can try it in the supermarket or on a bus, while you are doing the washing up or while you are chatting to a friend. Before long you will have impressive vaginal muscle power – strong enough to squeeze anything that happens to be inside your vagina.

Vagina (wet)

Many women complain that they produce too much lubrication and that when their vaginas are too moist neither they nor their partners can get proper satisfaction.

There is no cure for this problem I'm afraid. The only answer is to use a towel or strong paper tissue to wipe away the excess fluid.

Vaginal Bleeding (during or after sex)

A woman who notices any unexplained bleeding from her vagina before, during or after sex should see her doctor for an examination.

There are several possible explanations.

> The earliest sex orgies were organised for religious reasons – for the glory of God.

- If a virgin has had sex for the first time her hymen may have been torn – causing almost inevitable bleeding.
- If your partner has been rough then he may have caused some bleeding – particularly if your vagina was not properly lubricated before sex began.
- In post-menopausal women the vagina's ability to lubricate itself diminishes considerably.
- Bleeding may occur if the woman's cervix is damaged or inflamed.

Vaginismus

The majority of women who have never had sex before are nervous and apprehensive. When they see an erect penis for the first time they wonder how on earth it is going to fit inside them. They have no idea just how capacious the female vagina can become and the prospect seems daunting. Things may be made worse by the fact that they expect sex to be painful – either because they have read something suggesting that it always is, or because they have been told to expect their first sexual experience to be at best unpleasant and at worst painful.

Normally, the vagina is extremely flexible. However narrow it may seem to be it can quickly and readily expand to cope with the thickest penis.

But if the muscles around the vagina are tense the vagina will not expand and penetration will be so painful as to be impossible. This condition – known as vaginismus – is widely regarded as the female equivalent of impotence.

When the male partner tries to insert his penis into the 'nervous' vagina he invariably makes things worse. The more he pushes the more the vaginal muscles contract and the more impossible the task becomes. The anxiety creates more muscle spasm and the muscle spasm makes penetration painful and the pain creates more

---

A woman's breasts expand by up to one quarter when she is sexually aroused.

anxiety. What probably started out as a slight discomfort soon becomes a severe and raging pain and vaginal muscle spasms soon ensure that the penis does not enter the vagina at all.

Sometimes the fear of pain is only part of the story, for sometimes it is supplemented by a feeling that sex is somehow wrong.

Cultural and religious and parental pressures may conspire to persuade a woman that what she is doing is wrong. These feelings are particularly likely to develop if, for any reason, the sexual relationship is accompanied by any feelings of guilt.

It is worth remembering at this point that although vaginismus in virgins is usually psychological there can be physical causes. Any virgin who finds sexual intercourse painful or impossible should ask her own doctor for a check-up to make sure, for example, that there is no unbroken hymen.

Although vaginismus is a condition which most commonly affects virgins it can affect women who are sexually experienced. When this happens there can be several reasons.

First, there are the physical causes.

- An infection may make intercourse painful.
- Hormonal changes (such as those which take place during the menopause) may mean that there is relatively little lubrication inside the vagina.
- A scar may have developed after a woman has had a baby. Or if a woman suffered a tear after giving birth the repair may have been done clumsily with the result that there is genuinely insufficient room left for a penis to enter. (Sometimes, after giving birth, a woman who has had a number of babies and who has an unusually lax vagina may encourage the surgeon performing the repair to 'tighten things up a bit' – and his over enthusiastic interpretation of her request may lead to problems).

To make sure that there are no physical causes for vaginismus it is wise to seek a medical opinion.

The Vatican library is reported to contain 25,000 books on sex.

Second, there are the psychological causes of vaginismus in sexually experienced women:

- A married woman who is having sex with a new lover may feel guilty – and her guilt may turn into vaginal muscle spasm. It is not at all uncommon for a woman to be relaxed and perfectly capable of sex with one partner but to be tense and tight with another. Strangely, perhaps, a woman may be perfectly capable of having sex with her lover but quite incapable of having sex with her husband.
- A sexually experienced woman who is anxious to please her lover may be so tense and nervous that her vaginal muscles go into spasm and cannot easily be relaxed.

There are two things that any woman can do to rebuild her confidence and to conquer her problem.

The first thing she should do is to take the pressure off herself by agreeing (with her partner) not to try to make love for six weeks or so. Both partners should cuddle and touch one another and, if the relationship is a new one, try to get used to being naked with one another. She should get used to looking at and touching his penis. Mutual masturbation is an excellent way to get rid of some initial fears and anxieties while finding some immediate short term satisfaction. The important thing is that the process should not be rushed. The more nervous she is the more slowly and gently she should take things.

Next, she should gradually get used to the idea of having something inside her vagina by trying this simple exercise:

1. Make sure that you will not be disturbed, and undress. It's a good idea to make sure that the room is warm beforehand since you will find it nigh on impossible to relax properly in a cold room.
2. Lie down flat on your back on your bed and raise your knees up into the air so that your feet are flat on the bed. Put a pillow

---

One in three women regularly fake orgasms during sex.

under your bottom to improve the angle of approach.

3. Wet the tip of your (clean) index finger with a little saliva.

4. Very, very gently push the tip of your finger into your vagina. Be very gentle. There is no need to hurry. If it hurts – stop. Stop when you are convinced that you cannot get your finger any further inside.

5. Continue this exercise the following day – but try to get your finger a little further inside you.

6. Repeat the exercise every day until you can get your finger right inside you. Remember to wet it each time with saliva. If you prefer you can use a little baby oil.

7. Once you are happy that you can get a finger inside your vagina try with a tampon. Take the tampon out of its cardboard applicator and smear the end with baby oil or saliva. Then slowly push the tampon into your vagina in exactly the same way that you pushed your finger inside.

8. Once you can do this fairly easily and comfortably try deliberately tightening up your vaginal muscles before you push the tampon inside yourself. Make your vaginal muscles as tight as you can and then put the tampon up against the entrance to your vagina. You will probably find that you cannot get the tampon inside. You'll probably find that you can't even get a finger inside. Now, deliberately relax the muscles that you have tightened. And as you do so bear down as though you were trying to push something out of your vagina. This movement will help you to relax and open up your vaginal muscles. While you are relaxing deliberately push the tampon into your vagina.

9. At this stage most experts recommend that you start using proper vaginal dilators. These are usually made of glass and look rather like test tubes (though they are solid). A set will

---

Some male porn film stars can have erections and ejaculate at will.

consist of very thin dilators and quite thick ones. You should be able to borrow a set through your own doctor or gynaecologist. You use the dilators in exactly the same way as you used the tampon – starting with the thinnest and working your way up to the thickest. If you cannot get hold of a set of graduated dilators try using your fingers. Instead of using just one finger try using two. When you can get two fingers into your vagina without any pain or discomfort try using three.

10. Once you have more confidence you can ask your partner to help you. Instead of using your fingers try allowing him to put his (clean) finger(s) inside you. Remember that you are still in charge – you decide how many fingers are used and how far they go in. (As an alternative to lying flat on the bed you may prefer to lie towards the edge of the bed with your legs dangling down and your feet flat on the floor. Your partner can then kneel down in front of you). Do remember that lubrication is vital and that if you haven't got anything else saliva is both safe and effective (assuming, of course, that there is no oral infection). Some male partners may be willing to prepare the vagina by applying the saliva direct from their own mouths.

11. Once the six week rest period is over – and as long as you are happy that your vagina can now accommodate at least two fingers at a time – you can try intercourse again. Don't rush. If you think you need longer then wait. Try to get yourself as relaxed as possible before trying. Make sure that the room is warm and that you use plenty of lubricant. And take things slowly. If sex is still impossible don't worry. You probably still need more practise.

The first bra was designed by a woman who wanted to cover up love bites made by her lover.

Vulva

The visible sexual parts of a woman are known collectively as the vulva.

At the upper end of the vulva is an area known as the mons veneris or mount of Venus, which is named after the Roman goddess of love. The mons is made of a pad of fat which covers the hard pubic bone and acts as a cushion during intercourse and is covered with a luxurious growth of tightly curled pubic hair which also has a cushioning effect.

Below the mount of Venus the two outermost parts of the vulva are the labia majora, the outer lips of the vagina. These are made of elongated rolls of fat and are regarded as the female equivalent of the male scrotum. Like the mount of Venus they are also normally covered with pubic hair. It is a fact of life but of virtually no practical significance that the left labia majora is usually slightly larger than the right one.

Inside these two large, outer lips are the rather smaller, inner labia minora – delicate folds of skin which are usually free of pubic hair and which run parallel to the outer lips. These inner lips are normally closed together to seal the vagina off from the world. As with the labia majora the inner lips are often of different sizes. The colour of the inner lips often changes from a pale pink to a darker, rather rich, royal purple when their owner is sexually aroused. In some parts of the world a large pair of labia minora are considered to be the essence of true beauty.

The gap between the two inner lips is known as the vestibule – rather appropriately named since it is the entrance to the vagina – and just above the vestibule and underneath the mount of Venus the two inner lips meet, splitting into two to form a small, protective hood for the sensitive clitoris – the female equivalent of the male penis.

Two thirds of married women say that they would marry their husbands again. (But one third say they wouldn't.)

Warts (genital)

The incidence of genital warts is increasing. Like all warts these are caused by a virus. Transmitted by sexual contact genital warts can be found on the penis, around the outside of the vagina and elsewhere in the immediate area. Sometimes there may be only one or two small warts visible but occasionally huge warty growths can develop.

Genital warts can be burnt off, frozen off, removed surgically or painted with caustic substances but all these treatments must be applied by a doctor.

One in five women claim that they improved their marriage by having an affair.

For a catalogue of Vernon Coleman's books
please write to:

Publishing House
Trinity Place
Barnstaple
Devon EX32 9HJ
England

Telephone   01271 328892
Fax   01271 328768

Outside the UK:
Telephone   +44 1271 328892
Fax   +44 1271 328768

Or visit our websites:

www.vernoncoleman.com
www.lookingforapresent.com
www.makeyourselfbetter.net

Other books by Vernon Coleman

Bodypower
The secret of self-healing

A new edition of the sensational book which hit the *Sunday Times* bestseller list and *The Bookseller* Top Ten Chart.

This international bestseller shows you how you can harness your body's amazing powers to help you cure 9 out of 10 illnesses without seeing a doctor.

The book also covers:

- How your personality affects your health
- How to stay slim for life
- How to break bad habits
- How to relax your body and mind
- How to improve your figure
- and much much more

'Don't miss it. Dr Coleman's theories could change your life'
(SUNDAY MIRROR)

'A marvellously succinct and simple account of how the body can heal itself without resorting to drugs'
(THE SPECTATOR)

'Could make stress a thing of the past'
(WOMAN'S WORLD)

paperback £9.95

Published by European Medical Journal
Order from Publishing House • Trinity Place • Barnstaple • Devon EX32 9HJ • England
Telephone 01271 328892 • Fax 01271 328768

Other books by Vernon Coleman

Mindpower

How to use your mind to heal your body

A new edition of this best-selling book which explains how you can use your mental powers for improving and maintaining your health. Topics covered include:

- How your mind influences your body
- How to control destructive emotions
- How to deal with guilt
- How to harness positive emotions
- How daydreaming can relax your mind
- How to use your personal strengths
- How to conquer your weaknesses
- How to teach yourself mental self defence
- Specific advice to help you enjoy good health
- and much, much more!

What they said about the first edition:

'Dr Coleman explains the importance of mental attitude in controlling and treating illness, and suggests some easy-to-learn techniques.' (WOMAN'S WORLD)

'An insight into the most powerful healing agent in the world – the power of the mind.' (BIRMINGHAM POST)

'Based on an inspiring message of hope.'
(WESTERN MORNING NEWS)

'It will be another bestseller.' (NURSING TIMES)

paperback £12.95

Published by European Medical Journal
Order from Publishing House • Trinity Place • Barnstaple •
Devon EX32 9HJ • England
Telephone 01271 328892 • Fax 01271 328768

Other books by Vernon Coleman

Spiritpower
Discover your spiritual strength

This inspirational book will help you rediscover your life's dreams and help you fulfil your ambitions. Also includes:

- Find out who you are (and what you want)
- Three words that can change your life
- How to get what you want out of life
- Use your imagination and your subconscious mind
- Why you have more power than you think you have
- How you can control your own health
- Why you shouldn't be afraid to be a rebel
- How to stand up for yourself
- Know your fears and learn how to conquer them

What the papers say about *Spiritpower*:

'The final tome in his trilogy which has produced the bestsellers *Bodypower* and *Mindpower*, this is Dr Coleman's assessment of our current spiritual environment, and his prescriptions for change. He advises both awareness and rebellion, recommending ways to regain personal autonomy and fulfilment.'
(THE GOOD BOOK GUIDE)

'*Spiritpower* will show you how to find freedom and give meaning to your life.' (SCUNTHORPE EVENING TELEGRAPH)

'This is a handbook for tomorrow's revolutionaries. Dr Coleman offers an understanding of the society we live in, in order to show where our freedom was lost.' (GREENOCK TELEGRAPH)

paperback £12.95

Published by European Medical Journal
Order from Publishing House • Trinity Place • Barnstaple •
Devon EX32 9HJ • England
Telephone 01271 328892 • Fax 01271 328768

Other books by Vernon Coleman

Food For Thought
NEW, REVISED AND EXPANDED EDITION

Between a third and a half of all cancers may be caused by eating the wrong foods. In this bestselling book Dr Coleman explains which foods to avoid and which to eat to reduce your risk of developing cancer. He also lists foods known to be associated with a wide range of other diseases including Asthma, Gall Bladder Disease, Headaches, Heart Trouble, High Blood Pressure, Indigestion and many more.

Years of research have gone into the writing of this book which explains the facts about mad cow disease, vegetarian eating, microwaves, drinking water, food poisoning, food irradiation and additives. It contains all the information you need about vitamins, carbohydrates, fats and proteins plus a list of super-foods which Dr Coleman believes can improve your health and protect you from a wide range of health problems. The book also includes a "slim-for-life" programme with 48 quick slimming tips to help you lose weight safely and permanently.

' ... a guide to healthy eating which reads like a thriller'
(THE GOOD BOOK GUIDE)

'Dr Vernon Coleman is one of our most enlightened, trenchant and sensible dispensers of medical advice'
(THE OBSERVER)

paperback £12.95

Published by European Medical Journal
Order from Publishing House • Trinity Place • Barnstaple • Devon EX32 9HJ • England
Telephone 01271 328892 • Fax 01271 328768

Other books by Vernon Coleman

People Watching

This fascinating book examines the science and art of people watching. By reading the book and following its advice you will be able to:

- Understand gestures and body language
- Look like a winner
- Negotiate successfully
- Make people like you
- Avoid being manipulated
- Look sexy
- Survive on the street

'The ubiquitous media-doc has done it yet again, this time turning his talents for producing gems of information in rapid-fire sequence to the field of body language and private habits. Once you start to browse you would have to be a hermit not to find it utterly "unputdownable".'
(THE GOOD BOOK GUIDE)

'*People Watching* by Vernon Coleman explains everything you need to know about body language and also how to read individuals by their style of clothes and the colours they wear. There are tips on how to make people like you and how to be a successful interviewee. If you want to look sexy for that special someone or you just want to impress the boss you'll be a winner with this book'
(EVENING TELEGRAPH)

paperback £9.95

Published by Blue Books
Order from Publishing House • Trinity Place • Barnstaple • Devon EX32 9HJ • England
Telephone 01271 328892 • Fax 01271 328768

Other books by Vernon Coleman

How To Overcome Toxic Stress and the Twenty-First Century Blues

If you are frustrated, bored, lonely, angry, sad, tired, listless, frightened, unhappy or tearful then it is possible that you are suffering from Toxic Stress.

After three decades of research Dr Coleman has come up with his own antidote to Toxic Stress which he shares with you in this inspirational book. In order to feel well and happy again you need to take a close look at your life and put things back in the right order. Dr Coleman shows you how to value the worthwhile things in life and give less time to things which matter very little at all.

The book contains hundreds of practical tips on how to cope with the stresses and strains of daily life.

'Never have I read a book that is so startlingly true. I was dumbfounded by your wisdom. You will go down in history as one of the truly great health reformers of our time.'
(EXTRACTED FROM A LETTER TO THE AUTHOR)

'This book is absolutely outstanding ... it addresses a serious problem which up until now has not been identified or discussed in any meaningful way. If you feel you have a lot of stress being generated from outside your life, this book is an absolute must. Personally, I am going to get five copies so that I can put them in my lending library and lend them to as many people as I can.' (HEALTH CONSCIOUSNESS, USA)

paperback £9.95

Published by European Medical Journal
Order from Publishing House • Trinity Place • Barnstaple • Devon EX32 9HJ • England
Telephone 01271 328892 • Fax 01271 328768